FOUNDATIONS OF SURGICAL NURSING

Jane Forrest
S.R.N., S.C.M., H.V.

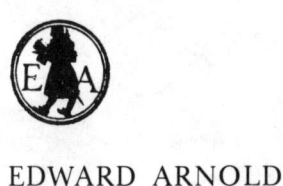

EDWARD ARNOLD

© Jane Forrest, 1974

First published 1974
by Edward Arnold (Publishers) Ltd.,
25 Hill Street, London W1X 8LL

ISBN: 0 7131 4235 9

All rights reserved. No part of this publication may be reproduced, stored in a retrieval system, or transmitted in any form or by any means, electronic, mechanical, photocopying, recording or otherwise, without the prior permission of Edward Arnold (Publishers) Ltd.

Printed in Great Britain by
The Camelot Press Ltd., Southampton

PREFACE

This little book has been written in the hope that it may provide a foundation of information on which the practical work on the surgical ward is based and to stimulate the nurses' interest in one of the most rewarding and satisfying aspects of nursing.

The emphasis here is on the day-to-day care of the patient, whilst at the same time providing facts that will help the nurse to link up causes with effects, leading to a greater understanding of the 'whys and wherefores' of the many interesting and varied occurrences in the surgical ward.

I sincerely hope that the nurses who read this book will find it helpful.

I would like to express my gratitude to my husband for his invaluable assistance in the preparation of the manuscript and the correction of proofs.

To the publishers I am indebted for their valued assistance and in particular to Miss B. Koster without whose encouragement this book would not have been written.

JANE FORREST

CONTENTS

		page
1	The Nurse and the Patient	1
2	Wounds	4
3	Healing of Wounds	9
4	Inflammation and Suppuration	12
5	Bacteria	16
6	Cross Infection and its Prevention	18
7	Specific Surgical Infections	22
8	General Preparation for Operation	29
9	Post-operative Care	38
10	Fluid and Electrolyte Balance	42
11	Blood Transfusion	45
12	Post-operative Complications	52
13	Disinfection and Sterilization	69
14	Ward Dressings	72
15	Surgical Emergencies	81
16	Care of the Elderly	86
A Short List of Surgical and Allied Terms		90
Index		91

1. THE NURSE AND THE PATIENT

As in every other department of the hospital, the patient in the surgical ward is the central figure on whom the work of the entire surgical team is concentrated. The surgical team in most hospitals consists of the Consultant Surgeon, the Surgical Registrar, a house surgeon, the ward sister, trained nurses and nurses in training. Every nurse, whatever her status, is an integral part of that team because she is in constant contact with the patient. She is the one who is in the best position to observe and to report any changes in the condition of the patient. The surgeon and his team rely on the nurses for accurate information on the daily and sometimes hourly progress or on any signs or symptoms or complications that may arise before or after operation. Equally important is the fact that it is to the nurse that the patient turns for comfort, courage and reassurance.

In the study of surgical nursing our first consideration is, of course, the man, woman or child admitted for treatment. In spite of vastly improved methods of anaesthesia and surgical procedures, the word 'operation' still induces fear in the mind of the patient. Fear of what? we may ask. To the nurse an operation is a matter-of-fact occurrence; something that happens to somebody every day. She knows the exact routine; why it is carried out and what is to be done for a particular patient. With increasing experience she knows the probable outcome of the treatment or operation. The patient knows nothing of all this and even in the unlikely event of a patient having some knowledge, it does nothing to lessen the dread of the unknown. For this is invariably the basis of pre-operative fear—the unknown. Whether the operation will be successful, whether there will be too much pain, how long before complete recovery or how the family will fare during his or her stay in hospital. These are but a few of the anxieties that may beset a patient's mind on being told that surgical treatment is necessary.

Fear gives rise to tension, which in turn lowers the patient's morale, with the result that he is less able to tolerate the anaesthetic and/or the aftermath of surgery. In short the degree of post-operative shock (p. 52) may well depend, to a great extent, on the degree of fear felt by the patient before or after admission to the surgical ward.

Such anxieties may be lessened considerably by the attitude of the nurses towards the patient. So often we are inclined to think that surgical nursing begins when the patient is prepared for operation, or more commonly, on return from the theatre. This is not so. It begins as soon as the patient enters the ward door for admission. It is from *that* moment that the skilful nurse will be alert to the mental outlook of the patient and to the existence of any underlying anxieties not immediately apparent to a casual onlooker. By her efficiency, combined with a cheerful, sympathetic attitude, the nurse can instil a confidence that will go a long way in contributing to the recovery of the patient.

Whilst considering the fear and anxieties of the patient, we must not forget those of the relatives, especially the parents of children and young people. They too may be in need of comfort and encouragement and will almost always turn to the nurse for reassurance; usually the nurse responsible for admitting the patient. Here a word of warning must be given. Very often the worried relatives, and sometimes visitors, will ask for information, including questions about the patient's present condition, the treatment to be given and the prognosis. The wise nurse will refer such enquiries to the Sister, Charge Nurse, Staff Nurse or other senior nurse in charge of the ward. No nurse, other than the senior staff, should ever express her own opinion on any professional matter regarding the patient. Too often such personal opinions may be misconstrued or, through lack of knowledge, may be completely false, to the distress of all concerned.

ADMISSION OF THE PATIENT

Patients are admitted to the surgical ward from a waiting list or as emergencies according to the urgency of the treatment required.

Emergency operations are carried out as soon as possible after admission in order to save life.

Major operations: the patient is usually admitted several days before operation. This gives the patient time to become accustomed to the ward and its surroundings and to become acquainted with the other patients and with the hospital staff. These factors are important to the welfare of the patient, especially after operation, because he will awaken to familiar sights and sounds around him and will therefore be more relaxed, an important consideration in post-operative nursing.

This pre-operative period also allows time for full investigation to be made into the patient's general condition and will include nutrition, blood pressure, urine tests, x-rays, blood counts and tests to establish the level of haemoglobin (Hb) and the blood group. (Where the Hb is below 70%, blood transfusions may be ordered to be given before operation (p. 45.) In some cases special investigations may be necessary according to the particular operation required. Physiotherapy may be carried out to include muscular and/or deep breathing exercises which will be continued after operation to assist recovery.

Information regarding any drugs the patient is taking at the time of admission, including their names and dosages, must be obtained. This is particularly important in cases where the patient's life is dependent on drugs, such as insulin, anticoagulants or steroids. Patients taking these drugs should carry a card stating the name and dosage of the drug. These cards should be attached to the patient's notes and the nurse in charge informed without delay.

The consent form for anaesthetic and/or operation must be signed by the patient. If the patient is incapable of signing, or is under age, the consent form must be signed by a parent or other responsible relative or guardian. The consent form must also be attached to the patient's notes.

2. WOUNDS

In considering surgical nursing there is often a tendency to relate it solely to the work of the surgeons in the operating theatre and to the ensuing ward dressings. Surgical nursing does, however, cover a wider range to include the vast amount of emergency surgery carried out in the dressing rooms and theatres of the casualty departments for the repair and treatment of many types of accidental injuries.

Before studying the methods of dressing wounds we will consider briefly some important facts relating to the various types of wounds. A wound is a break in the skin or mucous membrane or other soft tissues of the body due to operation or injury. Wounds can therefore be divided into two main groups: viz. *surgical* or *intentional* wounds which are *aseptic* and heal by first intention (p. 9) and *accidental* wounds caused by injury (trauma).

ACCIDENTAL WOUNDS

1. **Abrasions** are lacerations of the superficial layer of the skin caused by friction or excessive scratching from contact with some rough surface. An abrasion will heal more rapidly if, after gentle cleansing and the application of a mild antiseptic, it is dried and left exposed to the air.

2. **Contused wounds** are caused by a direct blow from a blunt instrument and are characterized by excessive bruising, the result of blood escaping into the underlying tissues, giving a bluish-purple colour to the surrounding skin. As the red cells break down and are absorbed, the dark colour gradually disappears. Where bruising is localized, the part is rested by the application of firm bandages or splints. For more extensive and generalized bruising with no severe injuries, a hot bath is

beneficial, followed by bed rest until pain and stiffness disappear.

3. **A haematoma** is similar to a contusion but larger blood vessels are involved. More blood escapes into the tissues forming a large, soft fluid swelling which in many instances causes considerable pain. A haematoma may be completely absorbed and disappear or it may become infected through a break in the skin. A similar collection of blood may occur underneath a clean cut wound, the swelling becoming tense and painful. The treatment is as for a contusion with rest of the part and the application of evaporating or cold compresses where possible. If it occurs under a surgical wound, several sutures may be removed to allow the escape of the collected fluid or it may be aspirated to relieve the tension.

4. **Incised wounds** are inflicted with sharp cutting instruments such as knives or razors and are not complicated by any tearing of tissues. The edges of the wounds gape and bleed freely because the blood vessels are cut. Added to this there may be risk of injury to other important parts of the body according to the depth of the incision made and the probable introduction of infective micro-organisms into the wound from the weapon used.

5. **Lacerated wounds** have torn, irregular edges caused by dragging or tearing forces such as moving machinery or fragments from explosions. Because the tissues are torn there is much less haemorrhage than from an incised wound, but there is greater risk of infection, particularly where large areas of dead or damaged tissues are present or where fragments of hair, clothing or other foreign material have been forced into the wound.

6. **Punctured wounds** are caused by pointed objects and include knife and gunshot wounds. The external openings are comparatively small but the wound may penetrate deeply into the body, causing injury to arteries, veins, nerves or internal organs. Foreign bodies, such as a bullet or shell splinters, or other contaminated material may be forced into the wound at the point of impact, increasing the risk of serious infection of the wound and surrounding tissues.

Small wounds are treated and, if necessary, sutured in casualty. Patients suffering from severe injuries may receive immediate surgical treatment in the operating theatre of the casualty department or may be transferred to a ward for further treatment or for more extensive surgery. X-rays may be taken in the x-ray or casualty department or with a portable x-ray machine after admission to the ward.

In all accidental wounds such as those described above, the risk of infection is an ever-present danger. The wounds may be either

(a) *Contaminated*, in which bacteria may have been introduced under the skin by the implement causing the wound but which have NOT invaded the tissues. This applies to the majority of accidental wounds.

(b) *Infected* or septic, where bacteria are present in the wound and the surrounding tissues are inflamed. Suppuration (the formation of pus) may be evident. Pyogenic (pus-forming) bacteria introduced into a wound may cause local inflammation, but if absorbed into the lymphatic system or the blood vessels may cause pyaemia or septicaemia (p. 13).

Where possible, accidental wounds are treated in the first instance at the scene of the accident by first aid means which aim at controlling any haemorrhage, preventing shock and risk of further injury and avoiding possible infection of wounds by the application of clean dressings or coverings to the injured parts.

On arrival in the casualty department the general condition of the patient is noted and where any signs or symptoms of shock or visible or concealed haemorrhage are apparent, immediate measures are taken to overcome these conditions. ALL wounds are a potential source of infection but the danger is much greater in accidental wounds, especially those contaminated by soil or horse manure in which the *tetanus bacillus* is prevalent. Where such contamination is suspected an anaesthetic is administered, the wound is opened up to be cleansed and any damaged tissue or blood clots are removed. In all cases of accidental injury, anti-tetanic serum is given intramuscularly as a preventive measure, unless the patient has previously been immunized against tetanus. Following the administration of anti-tetanic serum, the patient must be watched for 7–10 days for any signs of reaction to the serum. Signs and symptoms will include the appearance of an urticarial rash, headache, pyrexia, joint pains and albuminuria.

COMPLICATIONS OF WOUNDS

Shock, varying in severity according to the number and extent of the wounds and the amount of blood and other body fluids lost.

Haemorrhage which may be primary, reactionary or secondary.

Sepsis due to the entry of harmful micro-organisms into the wound.

Suppuration, the disintegration of the tissues and the formation of pus.

Sloughing occurs where the soft tissues over and around the wound are destroyed as a result of injury to, or blockage of, the tiny veins in the vicinity of the wound, preventing the efficient circulation of the blood to the part.

Necrosis means the death of a portion of tissue and may appear as an *ulcer*, when there is a loss of tissue on the skin or mucous membrane; as a *slough* when a piece of tissue is killed but not reduced to a liquid; as a *sequestrum* when part of a bone dies and as *gangrene* which means the death of the tissues of a large area of a limb or organ.

Surgical sinus. A sinus is a tract leading from a lesion deep into the tissues (p. 41).

Adherent scars which become fixed to deeper tissues, often to muscle tissue, causing a dragging pain on movement.

Keloid scarring is a condition where excessive fibrous tissue forms over and around the wound and, spreading into the surrounding tissues, causes the scar to become raised above the level of the skin in a dense fibrous mass.

Excessive contraction as in extensive burns where large areas of tissue are destroyed causing deformity or disfigurement. Contraction of the tissues may be prevented by the regular practice of movements and exercises as prescribed by the surgeon or physiotherapist. The nurse should be familiar with such treatment and its beneficial effects so that she can ensure that her patient regularly performs the required movements.

3. HEALING OF WOUNDS

Wounds heal in one of two ways:
(1) by **first intention** or primary union, or
(2) by second intention or **granulation**.

Healing by first intention occurs in clean aseptic wounds after operation or where accidental wounds have received prompt surgical treatment and converted into clean wounds. When the edges of an aseptic wound are brought together they will unite in a few days.

A blood clot forms between the cut edges and serum or plasma oozing from the wound 'glues' the cut surfaces together.

A thin layer of fibrous tissue forms between the edges of the wound into which a fresh supply of blood is carried from the surrounding capillaries.

A larger amount of blood flows into the surrounding area (inflammation). Where there is no infection this inflammation subsides in a few days.

This extra supply of blood to the part encourages the rapid growth and sub-division of cells which enter the blood clot to form new tissue.

Epithelium grows inward from the edges of the wound and eventually becomes scar tissue, completely covering and closing the wound.

To ensure the success of healing by first intention the following points are essential.

Strict asepsis must be maintained by the use of sterile instruments, dressings and equipment to exclude all risk of infecting a wound.

The wound must be protected from contamination from the air and from clothing by sterile dressings or, if left exposed, by the application of a 'liquid skin' spray.

Healing by second intention or granulation

This takes place under the following circumstances:

(a) where the edges of a wound have NOT been brought together;
(b) where there is any loss of tissue at the time of the injury, as in accidental wounds;
(c) where infection of a clean wound has occurred.

Healing by *granulation* is a long, slow process. The granulating tissue grows from the base and sides of the wound. Epithelial tissue closes in from the sides very slowly to form new skin. At the same time pus or serum is discharged from the surface of the wound. If a drainage tube has been inserted this must be kept clear of obstruction. Care must be taken to ensure that the drainage tube cannot fall out of position. Where the superficial growth of granulating tissue becomes excessive it is checked by the application of a caustic such as silver nitrate. Scar tissue formed from granulations is often large and unsightly and after contraction may cause disfigurement or deformity. Where the risk of such a complication exists, grafting of new tissue over the wound may be carried out by the surgeon.

RETARDED HEALING OF WOUNDS

There are various factors that may cause delay in healing, some of which may be foreseen. This is one of the reasons for the admission of the patient to the ward several days before operation. These 'delaying factors' may be due to the general condition of the patient or to some local condition on or near the wound and the surrounding area.

General conditions are those affecting the patient as a whole, such as anaemia, debility, malnutrition (especially where there is a lack of proteins or vitamins, particularly Vitamin C), jaundice, uraemia, pulmonary disease, advanced malignancy, excessive anxiety and old age.

Where wounds of the thorax or abdomen are involved, coughing, vomiting or abdominal distension may delay healing, as will the presence of a sinus or fistula leading from an internal organ through which digestive or other body fluids may drain on to the surface of the skin around the wound.

Local delaying factors may include infection due to pyogenic bacteria, non-pulmonary tuberculosis, inefficient drainage of a wound, foreign bodies, sequestrum (bone splinter), haematoma or deficient circulation of blood around the wound, especially in the extremities of a patient suffering from arterio-sclerosis. Also, where a wound has been sutured too tightly, where sutures are removed too soon or when the edges of a wound are turned inwards. Unless the cut edges of a wound are in close contact, healing is retarded.

To ensure satisfactory healing of any type of wound, the general health of the patient must be maintained by adequate fluid replacement, a nourishing diet, sufficient and adequate sleep and reassurance.

4. INFLAMMATION AND SUPPURATION

Inflammation is the response of living tissue to irritation or to interference that may be due to injury (trauma) or to infection and may be classified as *local* or *general* inflammation.

Signs and symptoms of local inflammation

Redness caused by the increased flow of blood to the surface of the affected area through the dilated blood vessels (arterioles).

Swelling due to an excessive amount of fluid escaping from the surrounding capillaries and lymph vessels into the tissues.

Pain resulting from the pressure on the nerve endings by the swollen tissues. Infection may travel along the lymphatic vessels to the nearest group of lymphatic glands which become inflamed and tender (lymphadenitis).

Heat arising from the acute chemical changes taking place and causing increased production of heat in the surrounding tissues.

Around wounds where no infection is present, as in a clean cut or surgical incision, inflammation is a sign that the healing process has begun. After a few days the inflammation subsides as healing is established (p. 9). The surgical nurse must be very sure that the inflammation seen in clean wounds does in fact subside and does not spread or cause undue pain or malaise. If the inflammation appears to be increasing in severity, the senior staff must be notified without delay because it may be a sign that the wound has become infected and infection of a surgical wound is a very serious matter.

Local inflammation that cannot be controlled in the early stages usually goes on to *suppuration*, i.e. the breaking down of tissue by virulent micro-organisms such as *Staphylococcus*, *Streptococcus*, *Pneumococcus* or *Bacillus coli* (p. 16).

The treatment of local inflammation is by the administration of antibiotics and, where possible, the application of heat to the area. Applied heat helps to bring more blood to the inflamed area and thus assist the natural process of healing.

GENERAL INFLAMMATION

Where infection becomes severe and cannot be controlled, harmful micro-organisms or their toxins invade the blood stream, causing a condition in which the whole body is affected and the patient may become seriously ill; an occurrence that every surgical nurse prays will not happen. Toxins entering the blood stream give rise to *toxaemia* and if the micro-organisms themselves gain entry and multiply, *septicaemia* occurs.

Signs and symptoms

Toxaemia: Pyrexia, rapid pulse rate, sweating, scanty urine which is highly coloured and very acid.

Septicaemia: Pyrexia, dyspnoea, bronchitis or pneumonia, albuminuria, haematuria, rigor.

Treatment

Chemotherapy, complete rest and copious fluids. The patient will need skilful and constant nursing care. The aim of such care is the alleviation of the symptoms as they arise, combined with close observation and reassurance of the patient.

SEPTIC CONDITIONS

An abscess is an extremely painful condition caused by a collection of pus in a localized area. Around this infected area is built up a barrier of living granulation tissue containing many leucocytes that prevent the enclosed pus from spreading into the surrounding tissues. When an abscess forms the pressure of the pus inside the cavity builds up and tends to force it into the area of least resistance. If the abscess is near the surface, the skin over the cavity will become stretched and thin and a yellowish area can be seen. This is called 'pointing' of an abscess. Eventually the skin will split allowing the pus to escape. When an abscess occurs internally a surgical intervention by incision may be necessary to provide an outlet through which the pus is drained.

A *stitch abscess* is a slight infection that may arise around a stitch or stitches, often due to bacteria being carried into the wound.

Pyaemia is a condition in which abscesses form in many parts of the body. Particles of an infected blood clot (embolus) from some septic focus, as in an inflamed vein, break away to circulate in the blood stream. These infected particles block the small blood vessels in various parts of the body, sometimes in the liver or brain. Wherever they lodge abscess formation takes place. Treatment is by drainage of the abscesses wherever possible combined with chemotherapy. Pyaemia is an extremely serious condition that may lead to extreme exhaustion and collapse.

Ulceration means the destruction of cellular tissue on free surfaces, covered by skin or mucous membrane. Ulcers may be classified according to the cause but, whatever the cause, all are invaded by bacteria and suppuration arises.

Traumatic ulcers are those caused by injury to the skin by bruising or pressure, as from plaster, splints or from sitting or lying too long in one position (**N.B.** a pressure sore is an ulcer) and by severe burns caused by excessive heat or chemicals.

Circulatory ulcers are due to impaired blood supply to a part, e.g. varicose ulcers. These are very difficult to heal because the edges of the ulcer become thickened with fibrous tissue. Occasionally excision of the ulcer may be carried out.

Trophic ulcers occur when the nerve supply to the skin is impaired by injury or disease.

Syphilitic ulcers are caused by *Spirochaeta pallida*. The ulcers may be multiple and run together and are accompanied by a very offensive discharge. Anti-syphilitic treatment must be given after diagnosis is confirmed otherwise they will never heal (p. 26).

Treatment

All ulcers, whatever the cause, must be dressed with strict aseptic precautions to avoid further infection. Antibiotics in some form are usually prescribed.

5. BACTERIA

Harmful bacteria, often referred to as micro-organisms or germs, are one of the smallest and simplest forms of life known.

With regard to their requirement of oxygen, bacteria are classified as:

(a) *Aerobic*—those which require air for their continued existence, and

(b) *Anaerobic*—those that can survive without air.

Under favourable conditions they are capable of rapidly reproducing themselves by division and multiplication of each cell. They have the ability to produce toxins that in severe cases of infection produce signs and symptoms of severe illness in the patient (p. 13). Some micro-organisms, however, are able to assume a protective covering in which they can remain alive but inert until conditions become favourable for their regrowth. They then become active and multiply. These temporarily inactive bacteria are known as *spores* and are difficult to destroy. A temperature of 130° C is required for their destruction.

For their continued existence micro-organisms of all types need nourishment, warmth, moisture and darkness. These conditions exist in the body and a break in the skin will provide access for the bacteria unless strict aseptic precautions are observed in the care of wounds or when carrying out any other surgical procedures, not forgetting the administration of hypodermic, intramuscular or intravenous injections.

Micro-organisms causing inflammation and/or suppuration

Staphylococcus pyogenes cause boils, carbuncles, abscesses, bone lesions, osteomyelitis, septicaemia and pneumonia.

Streptococcus pyogenes (Haemolytic streptococci) cause cellulitis, peritonitis, septicaemia, erysipelas and acute abscesses.

Pneumococci are the cause of empyema, pneumonia and sometimes peritonitis.

Escherichia coli (Esch. coli). This organism normally exists in the colon where it does no harm (non-pathogenic) but if perforation of the intestines occurs, *Esch. coli* may invade the peritoneal cavity causing peritonitis (p. 17).

Tubercle bacilli may affect the lungs (pulmonary tuberculosis) or glands, bones, joints, kidneys or skin (non-pulmonary tuberculosis) (p. 25).

Tetanus bacilli usually gain entrance to the body through wounds.

6. CROSS INFECTION AND ITS PREVENTION

Cross infection means the passing of virulent micro-organisms from one person to another. This is an extremely serious matter in any ward, but in the surgical ward it can spell utter disaster. Every member of the staff should be acutely aware of the dangers of cross infection but the onus of responsibility rests on the nursing staff. One careless or thoughtless action could prove disastrous to the work of the surgical team, causing severe complications and great suffering to the patient.

So what can be done to prevent this constant threat of cross infection? Primarily we must know where these harmful bacteria are to be found and how to prevent them from multiplying and spreading. This does mean that a very strict standard of personal hygiene must be maintained and that even whilst carrying out the daily ward routines, the nurse is constantly aware of the presence of harmful bacteria in the ward. Infection may be spread by direct contact from hands, bedding or equipment, by airborne bacteria, by dust and by flies.

Every nurse should wash her hands on entering and, for her own safety, before leaving the ward; before and after any nursing procedure; after personal toilet and, of course, immediately after handling bed-pans and urinals.

A nurse's hands are one of her most valuable assets of which she can be justly proud because they do so much for so many. They need and deserve the greatest care. After being washed and well dried, a suitable hand-cream should be used each time to keep the skin supple and to prevent it from becoming dry and cracked, especially in cold weather. Any kind of break in the skin, such as a cut or abrasion, is a potential source of infection to both nurse and patient and therefore must be covered immediately with a protective dressing and the matter reported to the nurse in charge of the ward who will decide whether that particular nurse may or may not carry out or assist with the surgical procedures on the ward.

The finger nails should receive the same careful attention because they form a convenient hiding place for harmful micro-organisms. They should be kept short mainly because long nails are a potential source of danger to the patients through accidental injury to the skin and the introduction of bacteria from under the nails and because, if they are long, the risk of a broken nail is intensified. Nail varnish should NEVER be used whilst on duty. The varnish itself may flake off to carry infection or may even fall imperceptibly on or near a wound. Nails that are immaculately clean and well cared for look most attractive and professional.

Hair should be neat and well controlled with no loose ends that hang over a patient because, here again, even the cleanest hair harbours a certain amount of dust and, therefore, micro-organisms.

Contamination can be carried by *droplet infection* (airborne) whereby micro-organisms are forcibly expelled into the air from the naso-pharynx and throat during sneezing and coughing or even loud talking. The micro-organisms are borne in the invisible spray of moisture expelled from the mouth to fall on the nearest object. The moisture dries and the bacteria are left. Unnecessary talking between nurses and patients whilst sterile procedures are being carried out increases the risk of droplet infection and should be avoided.

It is for this reason that face masks are used for ALL surgical procedures, but while wearing a mask the nurse should be careful to avoid touching it until she has finished because bacteria may be transmitted from the mask to the hands and thence to the patient. After use, masks should be thrown away with the soiled dressings; they must NEVER be put into the uniform pocket. Paper handkerchiefs should be used by everybody in the ward and disposed of immediately after use.

From the above notes it becomes obvious that any nurse suffering from a cold should report the matter without delay and visitors should be warned of the dangers of infecting a patient.

Bedding in a ward must inevitably become a trap for bacteria spread by airborne and droplet infection; great care must therefore be taken when making beds to ensure that harmful micro-organisms are not spread around. Every nurse should remember that surgical patients are at risk from infection at all times. Bedding from one bed must never be placed on another bed or allowed to touch the floor where it will certainly become contaminated. Sheets and blankets must never be shaken in the ward. Flapping the sheets over a patient not only spreads infection, it is uncomfortable for the patient and is quite unnecessary. The same applies to the pillows: a really good nurse can give a patient the correct support in the right places without thumping and banging the pillows which only serves to raise unseen clouds of bacteria-laden dust and fluff. Soiled linen should be handled as little as possible and placed into a carrier at the bedside immediately on removal from the bed. It must never be gathered up into the nurse's arms otherwise her arms and the entire front of her uniform become carriers of infection. After handling soiled linen the hands should be washed.

Sanitary annexes, together with all the equipment contained therein, must be kept scrupulously clean at all times. Bed-pans, urinals, sputum mugs and specimen glasses must be spotlessly clean. A tiny speck of excreta allowed to remain on any surface can, by spreading bacteria, do untold harm in the surgical ward.

For the sanitary rounds a nurse should wear a special gown reserved for this purpose to prevent contamination of the uniform.

Where possible disposable bed-pan covers should be used during a toilet round but should not be transferred from one bed-pan to another. After handling or using a bed-pan the patient should be given the opportunity of washing the hands.

Dust in the ward is loaded with harmful micro-organisms of all kinds. It is therefore essential that all bed-making, sweeping and dusting is finished at least one hour before ward dressings or other surgical procedures are started. Floors and high ledges should be cleaned by vacuum cleaners and sweeping kept to the minimum. The use of dusters dampened with disinfectant helps in preventing dust from being spread around the ward.

Flies are another hazard in the battle against infection. They carry the most harmful of micro-organisms in the filth on their feet and bodies which they deposit wherever they settle. Every effort should be made to destroy them with one of the many fly-killers now available. Mesh screens fitted to doors and windows should be kept closed. All food (including fruit) and drink left standing on bedside tables and lockers in the ward should be kept covered at all times.

Precautions against cross infection must be extended to the ward kitchen where the highest standard of hygiene should be maintained with full use of the refrigerator. No food, especially milk or milky foods, should be left exposed in the kitchen. Disposable paper towels are a great advance on the cotton and linen dish cloths and tea towels that soon become wet, grubby and odorous. These can harbour harmful micro-organisms that are easily transferred to the ward on trays, crockery, cutlery, etc. Constant watch should be made on waste food and rubbish bins to ensure that they are being put to their proper use and that they are closely covered with firmly fitted lids.

In the fight against cross infection in the surgical ward, continual and strict attention must be paid to the most minute details regarding social and surgical cleanliness by every member of the staff.

7. SPECIFIC SURGICAL INFECTIONS

A specific surgical infection is one caused by a particular organism as, for example, tetanus, which can only be caused by infection with the tetanus bacillus, and tuberculosis by the tubercle bacillus.

TETANUS (Lock-jaw)

This may develop as a result of the contamination of wounds by the tetanus bacilli. These organisms obtain their oxygen from the surrounding body tissues and not directly from the air (anaerobic). The tetanus bacillus usually develop in deeply punctured wounds but may occur in any wound contaminated with soil and/or manure. This micro-organism produces a powerful toxin which poisons the motor nerve cells of the central nervous system causing varying degrees of muscular spasm in those muscles supplied by the affected nerves.

Signs and symptoms

The incubation period is from 7–14 days after infection. The shorter the incubation period the more severe the disease. If under three days, death may occur in spite of treatment. Recovery usually takes place where the disease manifests itself after the 12th day of the incubation period. The first symptom is a general stiffness of the muscles, particularly those of the jaw. Muscle rigidity becomes obvious after 24 hours and in many cases the mouth cannot be opened (trismus). It is for this reason that tetanus is commonly known as 'lock-jaw'. As the disease progresses more severe muscular spasms occur with arching of the spine and the head thrown back (opisthotonos). Spasms of the sphincters of the body cause extreme difficulty in swallowing, micturition and defaecation. The greatest danger is spasm of the respiratory muscles leading to laryngeal spasm or long periods of cyanosis due to lack of oxygen (anoxia) resulting in death.

Treatment

Where contamination of a wound by the tetanus bacillus is suspected, the wound is excised and dead or damaged tissue or blood clot is removed. The wound is not sutured, the cavity being lightly packed with sterile gauze dressing to allow free drainage. Where the disease is evident, the patient is nursed in an isolated dark room or in the Intensive Care Unit. Absolute quiet must be maintained because the disease severely affects the central nervous system. Sudden movements, loud noises or bright light invariably cause the violent spasms so dreaded by the patient. Oxygen must be kept readily available and, in severe cases, an intubation tray with suitable endotracheal tubes and attachments for immediate use in an emergency should be close at hand. Tracheotomy may become necessary where severe spasm (trismus) interferes with breathing (dysphagia).

Routine nursing care must be carried out as smoothly and quietly as possible and nurses caring for a patient suffering from tetanus must be very sure that their hands are warm before touching the patient: cold hands, cold water and equipment or draughts will induce muscular spasms.

Nothing is given by mouth. Intravenous fluids are given, with strict recording of fluid intake and output. The patient must be watched for any signs of either oedema or dehydration.

Always remember that the patient is very frightened and needs constant reassurance and although he may be in spasm and his eyes may be covered to exclude light, he can hear and understand all that is said by people in the room but cannot express his feelings.

Measures taken to prevent tetanus (prophylaxis)

The incidence of tetanus has been greatly reduced since the introduction of preventive immunization during childhood. Where a patient has not been immunized against the disease, anti-tetanus serum may be prescribed to be given intramuscularly.

GAS GANGRENE

This is the death of tissue that remains attached to the living body. It is the result of infection of a deep wound, particularly where the blood supply to a large muscle has been impaired or where there is complete obstruction of the arterial blood supply to a muscle. A tourniquet left in position for too long will obstruct the blood supply, as will a plaster splint that becomes too tight. The two main organisms causing gas gangrene are *Clostridium welchi* and *Clostridium sporogenes*, both anaerobic organisms found in soil or stable manure. They destroy body tissues and produce carbon dioxide and hydrogen gases around the affected area and a particularly virulent toxin that circulates in the blood stream.

Signs and symptoms

The patient becomes very ill with pyrexia, rapid pulse, low blood pressure and vomiting. The wound and surrounding tissues become dark, greenish and oedematous. The swollen tissues crackle with gas bubbles when touched. *Anuria* (suppression of urine) may intervene.

Treatment

The patient is isolated to prevent infection spreading to other patients and is nursed as for any severe illness. Infected tissues are excised from the wound which is then left open to heal by granulation and the dressings changed daily. Intensive chemotherapy may be ordered.

ERYSIPELAS

This is an acute inflammatory infectious disease of the skin caused by the haemolytic streptococcus (a micro-organism having the power to destroy red blood cells). This organism usually gains entry through a small wound or abrasion. Any area of the body may be affected but it is often seen on the face which becomes red, hot and painful. The inflamed area is raised above the surrounding skin and has a well defined edge. Later small vesicles appear spreading over the erythematous area. Where the loose tissues of the eyelids are affected, considerable oedema occurs and the patient is unable to open the eyes. The onset is sudden and the general signs and symptoms include headache, pyrexia, malaise and rigor.

Treatment

Routine nursing care as for any pyrexial condition. Affected eyelids should be cleansed regularly. Chemotherapy rapidly controls the infection and prevents it from spreading. Erysipelas is contagious and nurses attending the patient must be extremely careful to wash their hands thoroughly before touching another patient.

CELLULITIS

This is due to the direct spread of streptococcal infection into the tissues, especially the subcutaneous layers. The affected area becomes red, swollen and tender with severe throbbing pain. Pus may form but with antibiotic therapy the tissues will usually return to normal.

PYAEMIA

This condition is described on p. 14.

SURGICAL TUBERCULOSIS

Tuberculosis is an infectious disease due to *Myobacterium tubercle bacillus* which invades body tissues causing them to become inflamed, damaged or destroyed.

Human tubercle bacilli can be spread
   (a) by *inhalation* of the bacteria in air contaminated by droplet infection coughed and exhaled by infected persons. *Myobacterium* tubercle bacilli spread by these means usually cause pulmonary tuberculosis but may also affect other organs.
   (b) by *ingestion* through drinking milk from infected cows. Bovine tubercle bacilli enter the gastro-intestinal tract and commonly affect the mesenteric glands (the mesentery is the fold of peritoneum connecting the intestines to the posterior abdominal wall) or the cervical

glands in the neck. This type of tuberculosis is now almost eradicated by constant supervision and control of dairy herds and the pasteurization of all milk.

(c) by *inoculation* through a break in the skin and although this is now a rare occurrence, the danger of infection must be kept in mind in surgical nursing.

Surgical intervention may become necessary to effect a cure as in lesions of bones, joints or the partial or complete excision of an organ.

VENEREAL DISEASES

Syphilis and gonorrhoea are the two most common and dangerous venereal diseases which should be treated as early as possible. If neglected, they produce extremely serious complications in later life which may affect any part of the body. These diseases are spread by direct contact, mainly as a result of sexual intercourse between affected persons, but can also be spread by contact with contaminated linen or other articles used by infected persons. Nurses should be extremely careful when carrying out nursing duties for an infected patient. Gloves should be worn to protect the hands and, whilst wearing them, nothing should be touched beyond the confines of the patient's bed. After use the gloves should be washed whilst still on the hands, then sterilized immediately or discarded. The hands should then be washed equally thoroughly before proceeding with other duties.

Syphilis

This disease, caused by the *Treponema pallidum*, may be *acquired* as above or may be *congenital*, i.e. inherited from the mother during pregnancy. Untreated acquired syphilis occurs in three stages.

The primary stage. The initial lesion develops into a septic sore or ulcer called a *chancre* which is highly infectious. The primary sore disappears in a few weeks.

The secondary stage. This stage may occur before the primary sore disappears or from two to six months afterwards and indicates a general infection of the whole body. Any of the following signs and symptoms may appear: sore throat, ulcerated tonsils, sores in the mouth, a copper-coloured nonirritating rash, particularly on the face and back, loss of hair, enlarged lymphatic glands, anaemia and large wart-like masses around the anus and genital organs (condylomata). During the secondary stage, when the whole body is infected, all secretions and discharges carry infection. This fact must be kept in mind during surgical treatment.

The tertiary stage. The symptoms of advanced disease may appear from 2 to 10 years from the onset. In this last stage the disease may attack any organ of the body causing large, soft tumours called gummata. The skin, mucous membrane, periosteum, liver or central nervous system may be affected. Death may occur from chronic disease of the nervous or circulatory systems.

Congenital syphilis is not usually evident at birth but signs of the disease may develop in the first two weeks of life or later in childhood. Early signs include wasting of the body, the typical copper-coloured rash of the second stage, inflammation of the bones, snuffles with profuse nasal discharge or enlargement of the liver or spleen. Later symptoms are thickening of the cornea leading to blindness, a depressed bridge of the nose from destruction of the nasal septum, changes in the internal ear leading to deafness, notched upper incisor teeth (known as Hutchinson's teeth), nervous symptoms and cerebral deterioration. Congenital syphilis may be prevented by a full course of treatment given to the mother up to the twenty-eighth week of pregnancy. Antibiotics have been found to be effective in the treatment of the disease and are now used extensively.

Gonorrhoea

This is the venereal disease caused by the *gonococcus* which may infect the mucous membrane of the genital organs. In the male it causes a purulent discharge from the urethra accompanied by painful micturition. In women the cervix of the uterus and the urethra are commonly affected with purulent discharge from the vagina.

Complications in the male include inflammation of the testes (orchitis) and stricture or obstruction of the urethra. In the female, inflammation of the fallopian tubes (salpingitis), peritonitis or sterility may develop. Gonococcal arthritis or heart disease may affect both sexes.

OPHTHALMIA NEONATORUM

This is inflammation of the conjunctiva in the newborn which may be the result of infection by the gonococcus at birth. It is a serious condition which, if untreated, may cause blindness. Close observation is made during the first few weeks of life for any sign of redness or of discharge from the eyes. Should these symptoms arise, the baby is isolated, the doctor is notified and treatment started without delay. Irrigation of the eyes, installation of special drops or the administration of antibiotics may be ordered.

In surgical nursing the presence of a venereal infection, whether concealed or apparent, has an important bearing on the progress of the patient because the disease delays the healing of wounds. Extreme care must be taken to avoid the spread of infection.

For many of the infective conditions described in this chapter, chemotherapy is given as part of the treatment to overcome the infection.

Chemotherapy means the treatment of inflammatory and septic conditions by certain drugs (antibiotics) that destroy virulent micro-organisms and/or prevent their growth. Occasionally a patient is unable to tolerate one or other of the antibiotics, especially penicillin to which he may be allergic, and a rash may develop at the site of the injection (urticaria) with pyrexia. Patients who suffer from hay fever, asthma or eczema are most likely to develop signs of sensitivity to penicillin.

Nurses should wear gloves when giving antibiotics by injection to avoid the risk of a skin reaction. The penicillin types and streptomycin can each cause urticaria with irritation of the skin which can be most unpleasant. When expelling air from a syringe the needle should be kept in the bottle: if drops are sprayed into the air they may fall on the skin of the arms or face with the same result.

8. GENERAL PREPARATION FOR OPERATION

The detail of the preparation of patients for operation may differ somewhat according to the condition of the patient and the type and site of operation but the general principles are the same. The extent of the necessary investigations may be considerably varied; a fact which adds further interest to surgical nursing. You may ask why and for what reason these investigations are carried out and the answer to this question will lead you along an interesting path of research. Many anatomical, physiological and psychological facts concerning the patient under pre-operative observation will come to light and for the intelligent nurse a great deal of invaluable knowledge will be gathered on the way.

The main objects in the general preparation of patients for operation are to ensure:

1. That the general condition of the patient is satisfactory.
2. That the skin is as clean as possible, especially over and around the site of operation.
3. That the stomach is empty so that the patient is less inclined to vomit under anaesthetic and there is no risk of the trachea being blocked by fragments of solid food.
4. That the colon and bladder will not discharge their contents whilst their sphincter muscles are relaxed under the influence of the anaesthetic.
5. That the patient has sufficient restful sleep and is not unduly frightened or anxious about any aspect of the anaesthetic or of the operation and its aftermath.

DIET AND NUTRITION

Gross overweight in a patient may increase the risk of post-operative complications, especially with regard to the respiratory system. Where obesity causes any degree of dyspnoea, the patient is put on a reducing diet prior to admission and under medical supervision until the surgeon is satisfied that the general condition is improved.

An undernourished patient is given a high calorie diet with plenty of proteins, vitamins and fluids. Extra nourishment is continued post-operatively in order to build up the patient's strength and resistance against infection.

GENERAL PRE-OPERATIVE TREATMENT

The pre-operative diet after admission consists of light, easily digested foods with very little fat and roughage.

Efforts should be made to persuade a patient to stop smoking before the operation because the smoke irritates the mucous membrane lining the upper respiratory system, causing mucus to collect in the bronchus and trachea. This may give rise to respiratory difficulties during and after the introduction of anaesthesia. A tactful explanation to the patient is usually sufficient to gain his or her co-operation.

On the day before operation the skin is shaved over and around the site of operation. This must be done carefully to avoid cuts or abrasions. Following the shave a bath or blanket bath is given and the skin well dried. Talcum powder must not be used because particles may adhere to the skin which later might cause infection of a wound.

An aperient may be ordered 48-36 hours beforehand. Enemas are not generally given unless the aperient has proved ineffective, in which case a simple enema will be given the evening before the operation. For surgery of the colon more extensive preparation may be ordered to include a rectal washout or colonic irrigation.

Sufficient *restful* sleep is always important but more so during the night immediately preceding the operation. Sedatives may be prescribed but the nurse should be alert to the amount and type of sleep these produce. The attentive nurse will be fully aware of any wakeful periods the pre-operative patient may have and be ready to give the encouragement and confidence often so sorely needed, remembering that 'a little comfort is worth a bottle of medicine'.

DAY OF OPERATION

An early morning specimen of urine is obtained, the amount measured and recorded and tested for albumen, sugar and ketone bodies. Any abnormalities found must be reported immediately and recorded on the patient's chart.

Preparation of the skin will depend entirely upon the wishes of the surgeon. In some hospitals it is the practice for the skin preparation to be started in the ward. The skin over the site of the operation is cleansed with surgical spirit or ether to remove any trace of grease from the surface, then painted with an antiseptic. The area is then covered with a sterile towel which is left in place until the patient is in the theatre. In other hospitals the surgeon may prefer to prepare the skin in the theatre immediately before the incision is made.

All jewellery, including wrist watches, should be removed and handed to the Ward Sister or Charge Nurse for safe keeping (it is wise to make a list of such articles before leaving the bedside). Wedding rings should be covered with a piece of plaster if they are difficult to remove from the finger. All hair pins and grips must also be removed. If the hair is long it must be firmly secured under a cotton cap completely covering the hair. Female patients with long hair should have it arranged in two plaits for comfort before tying on the cap.

All traces of make-up, including nail varnish, must be removed before going to the theatre because artificial colourings mask the true colour of the patient's skin and nails making it difficult for the anaesthetist to recognize or check signs of pallor or cyanosis in the unconscious patient. False teeth are removed to avoid any possibility of dentures impeding the administration of anaesthetic or blocking the trachea during anaesthesia. They should be put into antiseptic and placed in a safe place until required again. A mouth wash may be given which will refresh the patient: the nurse should stay with the patient to ensure that none of this is swallowed.

The bladder must be emptied immediately before leaving the ward for the theatre. If, through fear or nervousness, this is impossible, catheterization may be necessary. Before pelvic operations, catheterization of the bladder is always carried out.

The patient is then dressed in a special theatre gown fastened with tapes at the back for easy removal. In some hospitals long woollen stockings are drawn over the feet and legs for added warmth. Where stockings are not used the lower limbs are securely wrapped in a blanket.

An identity label must be attached to the wrist or ankle with the *full* name of the patient (initials must not be used) and the name or number of the ward. In many hospitals the type of operation and the names and dosages of pre-medication drugs are also included. It is extremely important that the name and age of the patient should be *exactly* the same as that on the patient's case sheet. This cannot be stressed too strongly because it is not uncommon for two people in the same hospital, and indeed in the same ward, to have identical forenames and surnames and serious accidents have occurred as a result of mixed identities. The responsibility must lie with the nurse escorting the patient from the ward to the theatre, that she has the right notes for the right patient.

The nurse taking the patient to the theatre must take with her a receiver or bowl and towel, mouth gag, tongue forceps, tongue depresser and sponge-holding forceps with a gauze swab firmly clamped in place. These instruments are in readiness for clearing the mouth in case of obstruction immediately after operation (Fig. 1). She must also take the patient's x-rays and notes including the consent form duly signed. If the consent form is not signed the surgeon must be notified without delay.

PRE-MEDICATION

The main reason for pre-medication is to allay fear and anxiety about the operation by making the patient relaxed and drowsy and to reduce secretions especially saliva and mucus in the upper respiratory tract and lungs.

A combination of drugs may be ordered by the anaesthetist to be given $\frac{1}{2}$ to 1 hour before anaesthesia is induced. Pre-medication drugs commonly used are omnopon with scopolomine, morphia with atropine or pethidine with atropine. The amount prescribed will depend upon the age and condition of the patient. When giving the pre-medication, the patient should be reassured by a simple explanation as to the general purpose of the injection and persuaded to relax comfortably in bed and to go to sleep. Curtains should be drawn round the bed and the ward kept as quiet as possible until the drugs have taken effect. If the administration of the pre-medication drugs is forgotten or delayed, the injection must be withheld until the anaesthetist is informed. This must be done immediately as the lapse of time between the injection of pre-medication drugs and the arrival of the patient in the theatre has an important bearing on the induction of anaesthesia.

The patient is covered warmly with the special blankets and

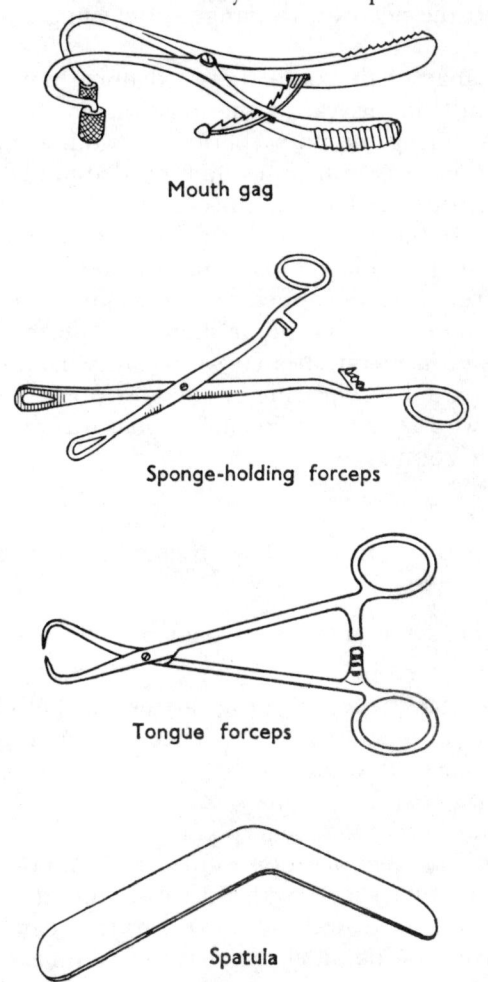

Mouth gag

Sponge-holding forceps

Tongue forceps

Spatula

Fig. 1. Surgical instruments

lifted by porters on to the trolley. The nurse must make sure that the pillow is so placed on the stretcher that it cannot fall between the handles. If this should happen the head of the unconscious patient will fall backwards and may result in severe injury to the cervical or cranial nerves. Strict watch must also be kept on the arms and legs of an unconscious patient to see that they do not jut out or fall over the edge of the trolley where they may receive injury from walls, doors or any other projection. An arm or leg hanging from a trolley may cause damage to the nerves with danger of ensuing paralysis of the limb.

In the anaesthetic room the ward nurse remains with the patient until the arrival of the anaesthetist. If the patient is conscious during this short period of waiting, the nurse can give the quiet reassurance so often needed at that moment. If semi-conscious, that reassurance can still be conveyed by a light touch of the hand. No discussion regarding the condition of the patient should be made until anaesthesia is complete. Even where the patient appears to be sleeping soundly, one can never be quite sure that he or she cannot hear what is being said. These considerations may seem somewhat immaterial but they do have a direct bearing on the post-operative progress of a patient who later may remember what was discussed in the anaesthetic room.

ANAESTHETICS

Anaesthesia means complete absence of sensation with loss of consciousness.

Analgesia is the absence of pain but the patient remains conscious.

General anaesthetics are drugs acting on the brain to produce a state of unconsciousness. They may be introduced by:
- *(a) Inhalation* of vapour gases such as ether, chloroform, nitrous oxide and cyclopropane.
- *(b) Intravenous injection*, e.g. pentothal.
- *(c) Rectal injection* or suppository, a method rarely used except for patients with eclampsia (fits that occur as a result of untreated toxaemia during pregnancy). Thiopentone or paraldehyde may be administered by this route.

General analgesia is produced by small doses of nitrous oxide or trilene gases as used in dentistry or midwifery.

Local analgesia is where the analgesic is given by injection into the subcutaneous or deeper tissues. Drugs used for local application include procaine (novocaine, planocaine) and xylocaine.

Spinal analgesia: a local analgesic is introduced into the cerebro-spinal fluid by a lumbar puncture.

Epidural analgesia is similar to the above but the drug is injected outside the dura mater surrounding the spinal cord and subarachnoid space. Whatever the method used, the nurse should be ready to assist in placing the patient in the correct position as required by the anaesthetist. For general anaesthesia the supine position is usually adopted. Should the patient become restless the nurse must gently but firmly control the upper limbs, keeping her own arms clear of the patient's head and thorax to avoid hindering the anaesthetist. The lower limbs can be controlled by holding one arm firmly across the patient's knees and gripping the edge of the trolley on the far side.

Where intravenous anaesthetic is being administered the patient's arm should be supported by the nurse until the needle is removed from the vein because any sudden movement may cause the shaft of the needle to break off.

Spinal or epidural analgesics are administered under strict aseptic precautions. The assisting nurse should wear a gown and mask. The patient is placed in the same position as for a lumbar puncture with the back against the edge of the trolley or operating table. The knees are flexed and the head bent towards them thus curving the spine as much as possible. The nurse can assist the patient in maintaining the correct position by putting one arm under the knees and the other behind the shoulders (Fig. 2). This is uncomfortable and rather frightening for the patient and every effort should be made to reassure and encourage him until the anaesthetist has completed the injection.

36 FOUNDATIONS OF SURGICAL NURSING

When the patient is fully anaesthetized and ready to be taken into the theatre, the blankets are removed and left in the anaesthetic room, leaving the patient covered with a sheet. Once again care must be taken to see that the limbs do not fall or jut out from the trolley or that the hands are not lying underneath the buttocks; this could cause injury from pressure on blood vessels or nerves in the hand. In the theatre the patient is placed gently on the operating table and placed in the position required by the surgeon according to the type of operation to be performed.

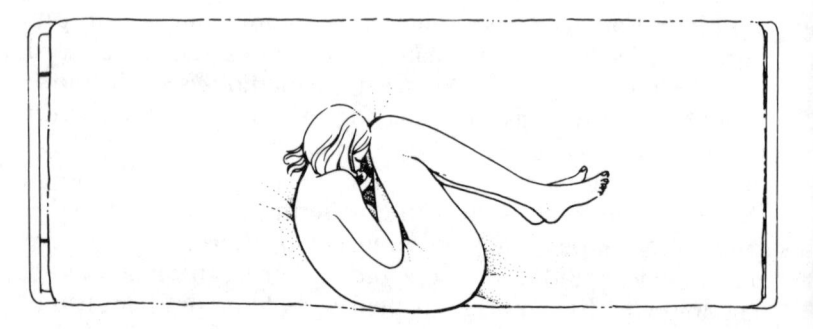

Fig. 2. Lumbar puncture position for spinal analgesia

The ward nurse may be instructed to stay in the theatre until the operation is completed in which case she could watch closely to see what is being done, e.g. the type of stitches inserted, the dressings covering the wound, any intravenous infusions given and the general condition of the patient throughout, so that she is able to give a report to the senior ward staff.

Before leaving the theatre precincts the following points should be observed:

1. The patient must not be taken from the theatre until the anaesthetist gives permission.

2. The patient must be gently handled at all times: rough handling may result in lowering of the blood pressure.

3. The patient must be warmly covered with blankets where the theatre is situated some distance from the ward or where, as in some hospitals, the journey back to the ward necessitates

taking the trolley into the open air, special care must be taken to cover the patient's head, leaving the face exposed.

4. Make sure that the patient's limbs are firmly secured inside the blankets so that they do not fall or jut out from the trolley.

5. Written instructions regarding immediate post-operative treatment should be obtained from the anaesthetist.

6. The tray containing the mouth gag and tongue forceps, etc. (p. 33) must be placed near the pillow on the trolley in case of emergency.

7. Where continuous intravenous infusion is being administered, the clamp holding the flask to the trolley must be securely fastened. Two nurses should escort the patient, one to control the intravenous infusion and one to watch the patient's general condition.

8. The nurse should be stationed at the head of the trolley where she can support the patient's jaw and observe any change in colour or respirations or any signs of vomiting.

9. If a pharyngeal airway has been inserted by the anaesthetist, this must not be removed until the patient begins to regain consciousness or coughs it out.

During transit from the theatre to the ward, the nurse is entirely responsible for the welfare and even the life of the patient who must not be left alone for one moment. The chin should be held up by gentle pressure on the vertical edge of the mandible on both sides. Should the patient become cyanosed or the breathing impaired the escorting nurse must stop and give her whole attention to the patient. These symptoms may be due to the tongue falling back and blocking the larynx. The mouth gag is closed and inserted into the side of the mouth, then opened. The tongue must be drawn forward until it is clear of the larynx. This can be done either by gripping the tongue on its upper surface with the tongue forceps or by pulling the tongue forward between gauze swabs held in the fingers. Any mucus or vomitus must be cleared from the mouth using gauze swabs clamped in the sponge holder. When breathing becomes regular and normal the forceps and mouth gag may be removed.

9. POST-OPERATIVE CARE

While the patient is in the theatre the operation bed is made up with clean linen, a mackintosh cover, one or two pillows and a small mackintosh over the head of the mattress. The bed is kept warm with hot water bottles or electric pads or blankets. *These must be removed on the arrival of the patient from the theatre* to avoid any risk of burns or scalds.

A tray is placed on the locker containing a small towel, a bowl of gauze swabs in water with which to swab the patient's mouth and face if necessary and a receiver or soiled dressing bag for used swabs. The mouth gag, tongue forceps, spatula and sponge holders are also left in readiness until the patient recovers consciousness.

Bed elevators or bed blocks, the 'drip stand' for continuous intravenous infusion and an oxygen cylinder should be at hand in case of shock or haemorrhage. Where spinal analgesia has been administered the foot of the bed may be raised for a short time to help prevent the severe headache that often follows.

On return to the ward the patient is lifted carefully into the prepared bed, making sure that all heating apparatus has been removed and, if still unconscious, is turned into the semi-prone position (Fig. 3) with a mackintosh-covered pillow placed firmly along the length of the spine to prevent the patient from rolling over on to the back.

CARE OF PATIENTS UNDER ANAESTHETIC

The immediate observations to be made are as follows:

Pulse: in the early stages of recovery the pulse should be recorded at $\frac{1}{4}$ or $\frac{1}{2}$ hourly intervals according to the condition of the patient. Note should be made of the volume, whether it is weak or strong; the rate, i.e. the number of beats per minute, and the rhythm, i.e. whether the beat is regular or irregular.

Respirations: whether quiet or noisy, moist or obstructed or if the breathing is dangerously slow. Difficult respirations may indicate the onset of pulmonary complications.

Colour: Healthily pink or whether pallor or cyanosis is evident. The colour can be judged from the lips, the finger nails or the lobes of the ears.

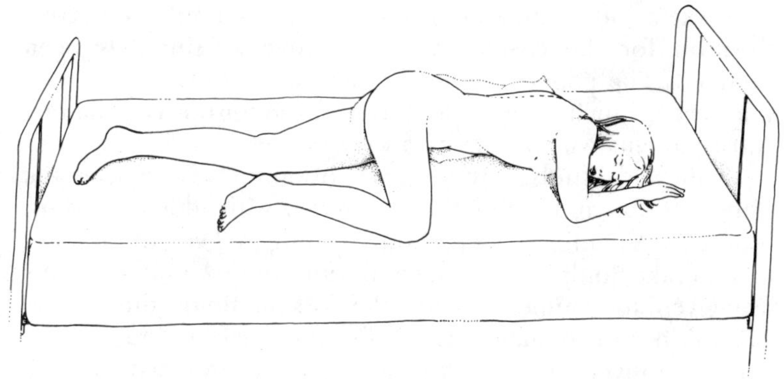

Fig. 3. Post-operative position for unconscious patient

Blood pressure: a low blood pressure may indicate the onset of shock or haemorrhage. If the systolic pressure falls below 100 mm Hg (millimetres of mercury) the nurse must report the reading. The doctor will be informed.

Skin: note whether it is warm, cold, dry or sweating. As long as the patient remains unconscious he should be turned frequently from one side to the other to prevent secretions from collecting in any one area of the body, particularly in the lungs. The legs should be moved gently to avoid the risk of venous thrombosis. All movements should be carried out smoothly and carefully (p. 61).

The unconscious patient must never be left alone and should be watched for any sign of cyanosis, extreme or sudden pallor, restlessness, shock, haemorrhage or vomiting.

NB. excessive post-operative vomiting at any time must be reported because this may result in severe loss of fluid and salt from the body (p. 56).

On recovering consciousness the patient may be moved into a comfortable position and given one pillow. The lips may be moistened (fluid by mouth is not encouraged at this stage) then left to sleep.

When fully conscious he is then washed, the theatre gown removed and replaced with the patient's own nightwear.

At this stage he or she should be encouraged to pass urine. One extra pillow may be given every hour until the correct position for the ensuing post-operative nursing has been attained. The patient should be persuaded to move the legs and feet as much as possible. If the reason for this is explained most patients will willingly co-operate.

If allowed, fluids may be given by mouth as soon as the patient is able to tolerate them, together with added vitamins, especially Vitamin C which aids healing. Where the patient cannot take fluids by mouth, continuous intravenous infusions are given to compensate for the loss of fluids during the operation and to maintain the fluid and electrolyte balance post-operatively (p. 42). Aspiration of the stomach may be ordered to prevent or control vomiting especially after gastric operations. An electrically controlled suction machine may be used for this. In some cases, aspiration of the stomach contents may be carried out through a Ryles Tube, using a 10 or 20 ml. syringe. Very often the tube is passed into the lower end of the stomach whilst the patient is in the theatre. The free end is strapped to the cheek. The syringe is kept in a bowl of water on the locker together with a measuring jug in which all fluid withdrawn is measured. The amount is entered on the fluid balance chart (see Fig. 4, p. 43).

In some hospitals the patient is transferred directly from the theatre to the recovery room where all equipment needed for the administration of oxygen, continuous intravenous infusions, blood transfusions and resuscitation apparatus is immediately available. Here the patient is cared for until completely recovered from the anaesthetic and in a satisfactory condition, then transferred to the ward. Visitors are not allowed into the recovery room unless death appears to be imminent.

POST-OPERATIVE CARE 41

The Intensive Care Unit is for seriously ill or injured patients in need of constant, skilled nursing care.

The ideal Intensive Care Unit is a large room with a clear floor space so that portable apparatus may be moved swiftly without obstruction. All equipment for saving life and for carrying out emergency procedures is kept in readiness, e.g. sterile trays for tracheotomy, intravenous injections or infusions, lumbar punctures and blood transfusions, portable x-ray machines, piped oxygen and electrically controlled respiratory, suction and aspirating machines and specialized monitoring machines.

The Unit is staffed by trained nurses with specialized knowledge of all monitoring and other electrical equipment and in caring for any emergency that may arise; accidental, medical or surgical.

10. FLUID AND ELECTROLYTE BALANCE

FLUID

Water is the basis of all body fluids and is the means by which the requirements of body tissues are transported to their destinations. In the normal individual about 60–70% of the body substance consists of water. This is contained both *inside* the cells (intracellular fluid) and *outside* the cells in tissues and in plasma (extracellular fluid).

Normal water balance is the amount of water in any form taken in from all sources and compared with the amount of fluid excreted or lost in any other way from the body, plus the insensible loss (perspiration and vapour contained in the breath), estimated at approximately 1,000 ml per 24 hours. This balance is maintained by the action of the antidiuretic hormone from the posterior lobe of the pituitary gland. In health the kidneys filter approximately 170 litres of fluid from the blood in 24 hours and of this amount 168·5 litres are reabsorbed by the tubules of the kidneys and returned to the blood stream, allowing 1·5 litres to be passed as urine.

ELECTROLYTES

Electrolytes or salts are inorganic elements which in water split into electrically charged particles called IONS. These ions are divided into two classes: alkaline (positive) known as CATIONS and acid (negative) called ANIONS, each electrolyte having an equal number of positive and negative ions. The chief electrolytes are potassium, sodium and magnesium which are cations (positive) and phosphate, chloride and bicarbonate, which are anions (negative).

The intracellular fluid with its electrolytes carries the essentials of nourishment. Normal metabolism tends to produce an excess of negative (acid) over positive (alkaline) electrolytes in the body, producing a tendency to acidosis. This is corrected by the production and excretion of acid urine.

Electrolytes determine the alkalinity of the blood and the efficient functioning of muscle tissue. Potassium has its main influence on cardiac muscle (too much can lead to cardiac arrest) while sodium and chloride influence the secretion of the right amount of water in the body.

The correct balance of water and electrolytes is of the utmost importance in the normal maintenance of the body or in recovery from illness. Injury or surgical intervention tend to upset the electrolyte balance, especially where there is any degree of shock or haemorrhage, excessive vomiting, gastric aspiration or intestinal obstruction. In such conditions the loss of water is accompanied by loss of sodium chloride with resultant depletion of sodium ions. Intravenous fluids are usually ordered to correct any deficiency of electrolytes. Electrolyte

DATE	TIME	ORAL	RECTAL	INTRAVENOUS Remarks	Amount Given	Gastric Aspiration	URINE	Other routes	REMARKS
	8 a.m.								
	9 a.m.								
	10 a.m.								
	11 a.m.								
	12 noon								
	1 p.m.								
	2 p.m.								
	3 p.m.								
	4 p.m.								
	5 p.m.								
	6 p.m.								
	7 p.m.								
	8 p.m.								
	9 p.m.								
	10 p.m.								
	11 p.m.								
	12 m'nt								
	1 a.m.								
	2 a.m.								
	3 a.m.								
	4 a.m.								
	5 a.m.								
	6 a.m.								
	7 a.m.								
	8 a.m.								
	TOTALS								INSENSIBLE LOSS 1,000 ml

TOTAL INTAKE   TOTAL OUTPUT

Fig. 4. Fluid intake and output chart

estimations are determined in the laboratory on specimens of blood plasma.

Herein lies the importance of the fluid balance chart; the amount of fluid lost or retained by the body indicates the increased concentration or dilution of the above substances in body fluids.

FLUID BALANCE CHART (Fig. 4, p. 43)

A very accurate fluid balance chart must be recorded. The fluid intake includes all fluids taken by mouth or by any other means including intravenous or rectal infusions.

Equally important is the output which must include ALL fluids excreted, drained, vomited or aspirated.

At the end of the day the amounts recorded in each column are added separately.

The balance of fluid is obtained by deducting one total from the other. Fluid lost in sweat or lung vapour cannot be measured. This is known as insensible loss and is estimated at 1,000 ml in 24 hours.

11. BLOOD TRANSFUSION

Normal human blood is classified into four main groups according to the factor or antigen carried by the red cells. These blood groups are designated as A, B, AB and O.

Groups A, B and AB cannot be mixed one with another because the serum from one blood group will cause the red cells of another group to 'clump', i.e. to form clots in the blood vessels. Should this occur the results could be fatal.

Group O blood does not react to other groups in this way and can usually be given without ill effect. Because of this, people having blood group O are known as universal donors.

There is another factor in the blood called the Rhesus factor that is present in 85% of the population and absent in the remainder. Where present the blood is said to be Rhesus positive (Rh+) and where absent Rhesus negative (Rh−). Rhesus positive blood must not be given to Rhesus negative patients because this would lead to a severe and serious reaction during transfusion.

CROSS MATCHING AND CHECKING

When a patient needs a blood transfusion, a sample of his blood is sent to the pathological laboratory to ensure that the correctly matched blood is used for the transfusion.

Attached to the neck of every flask of blood is a small, screw-topped bottle containing a few millilitres of the same blood as that in the large bottle. In the laboratory a few drops of this is mixed with a little of the blood serum taken from the patient and examined under a microscope. If no clumping occurs, the donor blood is reserved for the patient for whom the request was made. This is what is meant by *cross matching* of blood.

This small bottle must not be removed at any time because the blood it contains may be needed for checking with that in the large bottle during or after the transfusion.

The blood bottle has a large label stating the blood group it contains, together with instructions relating to storage and usage, the date of expiry, the serial number, the patient's *full* name and the name or number of the ward. At the bedside this label must be checked very carefully with the patient's case sheet and with the identification label on the wrist or ankle. Special care must be taken when replacing an empty bottle with a full one that the correct bottle is being used, especially if more than one transfusion is in progress at the same time, as often happens in a busy surgical ward.

It cannot be emphasized too strongly that the nurse has a great responsibility when handling blood bottles: mistakes can lead to severe and dangerous complications. It is therefore essential that strict attention is paid to the smallest details if tragedy is to be avoided.

When setting up a transfusion or changing bottles the labels should be checked by two people, one of whom should be a doctor or a trained nurse.

Changing the bottle

To change a bottle of blood, close the control clip gently without shaking the apparatus. The tubing between the clip and the intravenous needle should not be touched or blood may be drawn back from the vein into the needle. Place the empty bottle on a firm surface. Remove the outer cap from the new flask and take off the inner seal with *sterile* forceps. Transfer the stopper of the giving set from the old bottle directly into the neck of the new one. The glass tubes must not touch the outer surface of any part of either bottle or they may become contaminated and therefore unsterile. Open the control clip and adjust the flow. The rate of blood transfusion depends on the needs of the patient but is usually set at 40 drops per minute. The general rule is to give enough blood to maintain the systolic blood pressure at 100 mg. The patient must be watched closely with every fresh bottle of blood.

Empty bottles must never be thrown away: they are returned unwashed to the laboratory or blood bank from whence they came. They are unwashed so that any drops of blood left in them can be examined if necessary. This may be essential where a patient has shown signs of an adverse reaction to the transfusion.

Equipment for Blood Transfusion (Venepuncture)

Basic dressing trolley with sterile packs containing:

1. wool and gauze swabs, dressing forceps, gallipots;
2. 2 ml syringe and needle;
3. intravenous giving set (Fig. 5);
4. intravenous needles and canula.

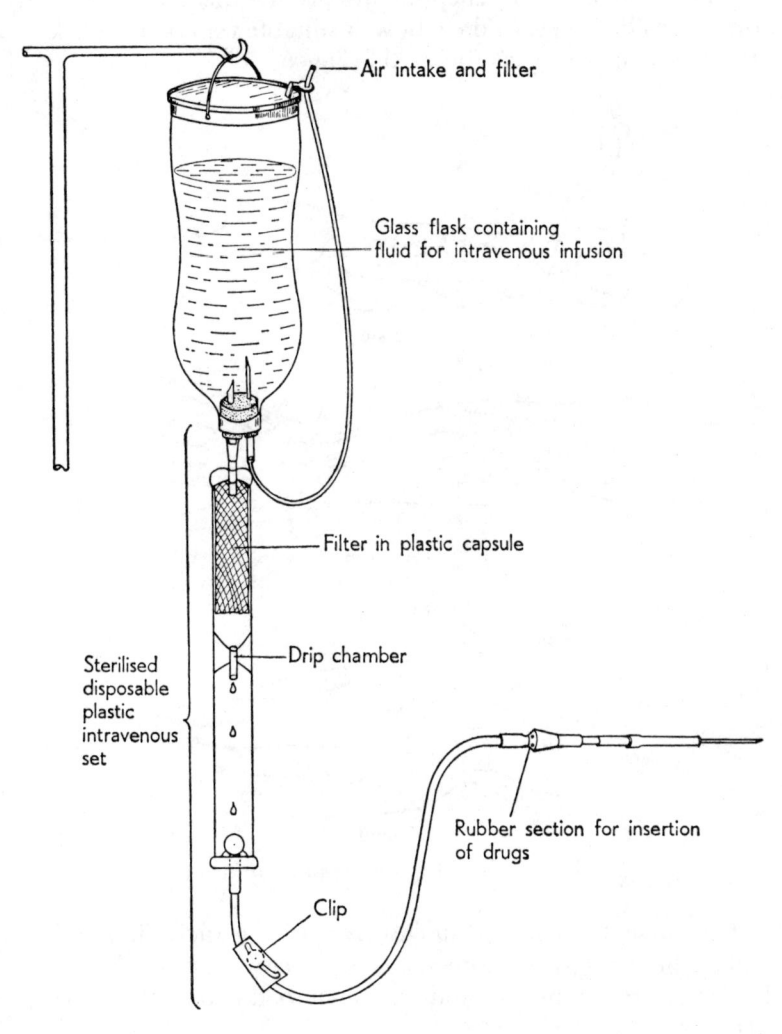

Fig. 5. Disposable set for intravenous infusions

Lotion for cleansing the skin.
Adhesive tape to secure the needle to the skin.
Covered splint to immobilize the limb.
Bottle of blood and drip stand.
Tubing clip.
Fluid balance chart.

The usual sites for venepuncture are the medial basilic vein on the inside aspect of the elbow, a suitable vein on the back of the hand or a vein at the ankle (Fig. 6).

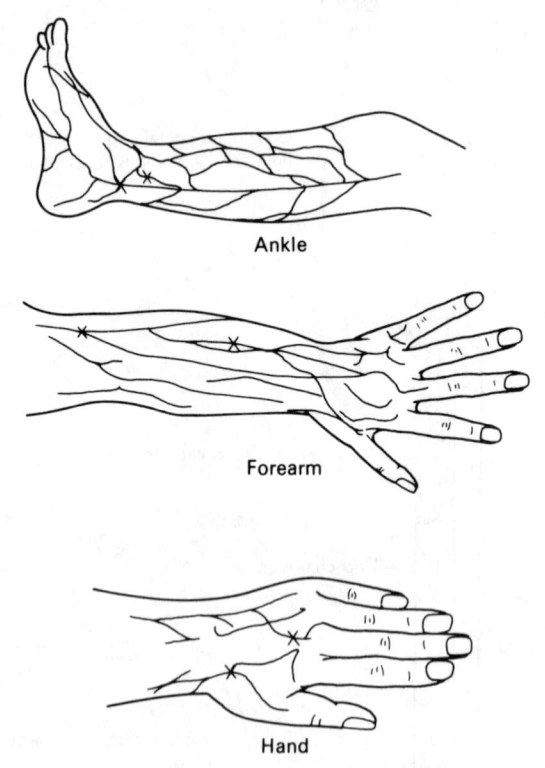

Ankle

Forearm

Hand

Fig. 6. Sites for intravenous infusions

The nurse will assist the doctor by applying and inflating the cuff of the sphygmomanometer as the doctor requires. After he has inserted the needle and canula into the vein the cuff is deflated.

The nurse should stay with the patient for a short while,

making him comfortable and giving reassurance but noting his general condition at the same time. Care must be taken to see that no tension is put on the tubing leading from the blood bottle to the needle. If the tubing is too long it should be fastened to the sheet with a large safety pin.

VENESECTION (Cutting down)

Where the blood pressure is too low to allow direct insertion into a vein, the surgeon may decide to cut through the skin to expose a vein. The vein is encircled by two ligatures using an aneurysm needle (Fig. 7). The ligature furthest from the heart is

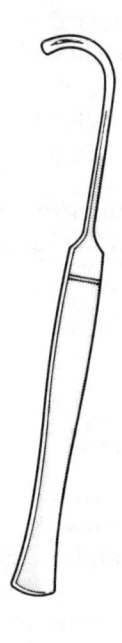

Fig. 7. Aneurysm needle

tied and an incision made into the vein with a small scalpel. This is a surgical procedure and strict aseptic technique must be adopted in the preparation of the trolley.

The equipment for the above procedure is the same as that for venepuncture with the following additions:

2 pairs of mosquito forceps;
small scalpel or Bard Parker blade in handle (Fig. 12. p. 80);
ligatures and sutures in sterile containers;
skin suture needles;
needle holding forceps;
local anaesthetic.

The drip stand should be so placed that it is continually in full view of the nursing staff but out of the direct line of the patient's vision.

The ward sister or charge nurse must be called if:
(a) the rate of the flow becomes slower or ceases;
(b) the intravenous needle slips or is pulled out (no attempt must be made to replace it);
(c) when one or two inches only of fluid are left in the bottle;
(d) if the patient shows signs of reaction to the transfusion.

Signs and symptoms of Reaction
Redness, pain or swelling around the needle area.
Restlessness, nausea and backache.
Rise in temperature.
Rigor.

INTRAVENOUS INFUSIONS

An infusion is the administration of fluids, other than blood, that are given to replace the loss of body fluids or as a means of introducing nourishment and/or drugs when nothing can be taken by mouth.

The fluids to be given intravenously are ordered by the doctor and written by him on the patient's case sheet. The necessary equipment for this procedure is as described for blood transfusion (p. 47).

Intravenous fluids which may be given are:

Sodium Chloride 0·9% (normal saline) to increase blood volume or to replace lost sodium.

Dextrose protein
Manitol protein } provide protein replacements as amino acids.
Aminosol vitrium

Dried plasma for shock, where there is little haemorrhage, to increase blood volume and contribute protein.

Dextran saline, a plasma substitute.

Ringer's solution, an isotonic solution containing salts of sodium, potassium and calcium.

Hartmann's solution is the same as Ringer's solution with the addition of lactic acid.

To the nursing staff of a surgical ward, the administration of blood transfusions or intravenous infusions are routine procedure but many patients (and their visitors) become apprehensive on seeing the intravenous apparatus, especially if blood is being given.

It is therefore important that during the pre-operative preparation an explanation should be given that transfusions are commonly given to assist recovery. Such reassurance will prove valuable in allaying any fears that may arise in the mind of the patient on recovery from the anaesthetic.

12. POST-OPERATIVE COMPLICATIONS

SHOCK

Shock is a condition in which the volume of the blood *circulating* round the body is lessened. This may seriously affect the vital organs, especially the brain or the heart.

Surgical or post-operative shock may be caused by pain or fear (neurogenic shock), chilling, haemorrhage, loss of other body fluids (oligaemic shock), or an obstructed airway or lengthy operation.

Signs and symptoms of shock

Pallor; cold, clammy skin; rapid, shallow respiration; faintness; low blood pressure.

Early recognition of the signs of shock followed by immediate and effective treatment may mean the difference between life and death for the patient. This is one of the reasons why an unconscious patient should never be left alone and why every nurse should be able to recognize the condition if and when it arises. At the first signs, senior staff should be notified without delay.

Treatment

Where the degree of shock is severe the foot of the bed is raised for a short time. The patient must be kept warm with a reasonable number of extra blankets. Hot water bottles should not be used unless placed on top of the blankets. Care must be taken that the body does not become overheated or further loss of body fluid as sweat will result.

The patient should be handled gently and made as comfortable as possible, avoiding too much movement as this may increase the degree of shock. The blood pressure will be taken frequently and recorded; the cuff of the sphygmomanometer should be left in place between readings to avoid disturbing the patient more than is necessary. As the degree of shock becomes more severe, the blood pressure falls but rises as the condition improves.

If the patient is conscious, the nurse should give quiet reassurance. There is no need to raise the voice because even a semi-conscious patient may hear, recognize and respond to the calm and confident voice of the nurse.

HAEMORRHAGE

Primary haemorrhage occurs at the time of operation and is dealt with in the theatre.

Reactionary haemorrhage occurs within the first 24 hours following operation *after shock has subsided* and the blood pressure begins to rise. As the circulation improves the blood flows with increasing force until it escapes from a weakened vessel not previously apparent. The nurse must be constantly alert to the danger of reactionary haemorrhage. The patient must be watched for any signs of haemorrhage and the outer covering of the wound inspected at intervals for signs of bleeding. This is especially important during the night following operation when the patient may be asleep or unconscious.

Secondary haemorrhage occurs *after* 24 hours and may be as late as 10–14 days after operation and is usually more serious. It may be due to sepsis of the wound or to a slipped ligature when a blood vessel contracts.

External haemorrhage can be seen from staining of the dressings and bandage covering the wound. The bleeding may be:
(a) *Arterial haemorrhage* from an artery. The blood is bright red and spurts out with every beat of the heart. This is an extremely serious occurrence and must be dealt with as an emergency. The medical officer must be notified without delay. Unless the bleeding is from the head, the patient is placed as flat as possible and the foot of the bed raised on blocks or an elevator. If the bleeding can be located, *direct pressure* with a

pad and bandage should be applied. Where this is not possible, firm pressure must be applied over the nearest artery supplying the area until help arrives.

In the post-operative care of amputations, a tourniquet should be attached to the rail at the foot of the bed but out of sight of the patient. An amputation bed is made so that the dressing can be seen by the nursing staff at all times. When a tourniquet is used it must be applied over a towel or clothing to give even pressure and prevent damaging the skin. A tourniquet must never be covered with bandages, bedding or clothing but should be seen clearly by all staff and must be released every 10–15 minutes and the blood allowed to flow freely for a few seconds. If this is not done the supply of blood to the tissues is cut off to a dangerous degree and nerves may be damaged with the result that gangrene or paralysis may occur in the limb below the point of compression by the tourniquet.

(b) *Venous haemorrhage* from a vein is purplish red in colour and flows in a steady stream. This type of haemorrhage may occur where the varicosed veins of a leg are ruptured. Such haemorrhage may be copious. The leg should be raised and a firm pad applied to the bleeding vein.

(c) *Capillary haemorrhage* is bright red and oozes out from the entire surface of a wound. Where this occurs post-operatively, it must be reported and the wound inspected at frequent intervals because it may be the forerunner of haemorrhage from a larger vessel.

Internal haemorrhage may be *visible* or *concealed*.

Visible haemorrhage from internal wounds may occur as:

Epistaxis from the nose. The patient should sit upright with the head over a bowl into which the blood is allowed to pour. Where the upright position is impossible the lateral position should be adopted with the bowl beneath the cheek. The patient should be instructed to breathe through the mouth. Blood clots forming a plug in the nostrils must not be removed.

Haemoptysis is bleeding from the lungs, the blood being bright red and frothy because it is mixed with oxygen. The patient should be nursed upright, well supported with pillows and encouraged to keep as still as possible. This is often difficult to achieve because the patient becomes very frightened and restless at the sight of the bright blood and needs all the help and reassurance a nurse can give.

Haematemesis is vomited in the form of dark brown granulated particles: nothing must be given by mouth.

Haematuria is blood in the urine indicating haemorrhage in some part of the renal tract. The urine may be bright red or cloudy in appearance.

Melaena is blood from the upper part of the colon excreted as large black shiny stools with the appearance of tar.

Signs and Symptoms of Internal concealed haemorrhage

Restlessness and anxiety.
Increasingly rapid pulse rate.
Gasping, sighing respirations or persistent yawning (air hunger).
Coldness and shivering with sub-normal temperature.
Extreme pallor.
Thirst.
Low blood pressure.
Faintness leading to gradual loss of consciousness and coma.
Concealed haemorrhage can only be detected by signs and symptoms. It is therefore extremely important that the nurse should have a sound knowledge of these so that she is able to recognize the onset of excessive bleeding and take immediate and appropriate action, remembering that post-operative haemorrhage and shock are frequently associated.

Where any degree of haemorrhage is suspected no time must be lost in notifying senior nursing or medical staff. This should be done swiftly and quietly, giving the patient no indication of the seriousness of the situation. The bed should be screened and the windows opened to allow as much oxygen as possible to circulate round the bed. If the suspected haemorrhage arises from the abdominal or pelvic cavities, all but one of the pillows should be removed with as little disturbance of the patient as possible. The foot of the bed should be raised on blocks or a bed elevator. For haemorrhage from the head or thorax the patient is supported in the upright position until help arrives.

PERSISTENT VOMITING

Most patients suffer a little post-operative vomiting which ceases after a short time, but persistent or excessive vomiting may have serious consequences because this leads to rapid and dangerous loss of water and electrolytes (salts) from the body (p. 42). Continuous vomiting may be due to the effects of the anaesthetic, particularly if ether or ethyl chloride has been used, or it may be the result of an intolerance to morphine that may have been given to the patient either before or after the operation.

Treatment must be commenced without delay to prevent the patient from choking or inhaling the vomitus. The pillows should be removed to lower the head and the patient turned on to the side. If unconscious, the nose and mouth must be cleared to provide a clear airway. To do this a tongue depressor may be needed to hold the tongue down to the floor of the mouth whilst the pharynx is cleared with gauze swabs held firmly in a sponge holder (p. 37). A conscious patient will need reassurance that the attack will pass. Meanwhile the head should be supported during the spasms and the face and hands sponged when the patient is able to relax for a few moments.

Drugs such as chlorpromazine (Largactil) 25 mg or cyclizine (Marzine) 50 mg may be ordered to be given intramuscularly to control the spasms. Where suction apparatus is available the stomach may be aspirated through a naso-gastric tube.

At no time must the patient be left alone as long as the vomiting continues. The frequency of the attacks must be timed and entered on the fluid chart together with the amount, colour and consistency of the fluid lost.

RETENTION OF URINE

This often occurs after abdominal operations especially where the kidneys are involved. It may be of purely nervous origin, aggravated by the difficulty of passing urine whilst in the recumbent position.

To encourage micturition the patient should be reassured that the retention is temporary. A calm, confident manner does a great deal in lessening the anxiety of the patient. As much privacy as possible should be given without giving a sense of isolation which would only increase the patient's doubts and fears. Where allowed, plenty of fluids should be given which MUST be entered on the fluid chart.

If no urine is passed within 8–12 hours the patient must be watched for signs of increasing pain and/or abdominal distension. Should this occur it must be reported to senior staff without delay. The doctor may give an intravenous injection of Carbachol which stimulates the muscles of the bladder to contract and so evacuate the urine. Should all other methods fail, catheterization may be ordered but only as a last resource and then under the strictest aseptic precautions because infection by this route is a very real danger.

ANURIA (Suppression of urine)

This is a rare but a much more serious complication that may occur following renal operations. It may also result from mismatched blood transfusions where the clumped red cells obstruct the tubules of the kidneys, or in severe shock where the blood pressure falls so low that the flow of blood to the kidneys becomes so inadequate that no urine is manufactured.

In order to check the amount of urine, if any, in the bladder, catheterization is carried out at regular intervals. No fluids are given by mouth and, because the mouth becomes dry, oral hygiene is important.

Where treatment proves ineffective, uraemia may intervene and the patient becomes dangerously ill.

HICCOUGH

This is a complication that sometimes arises after extensive abdominal or urinary tract operations. It is a spasmodic contraction of the diaphragm which may be due to stimulation of the phrenic or vagus nerves during operation.

Persistent post-operative hiccough can be distressing and exhausting. If a patient does begin to hiccough, close observation should be maintained on the duration of the spasms which should be reported if they become persistent or if the patient shows signs of distress.

Where the usual methods, such as drinking a glass of water or trying to control the breath, are ineffective, sedatives may be ordered to be given intravenously for rapid relief of the spasms or inhalations of a mixture of carbon dioxide and oxygen may be given by the doctor.

CONSTIPATION

Constipation is common after abdominal operations, usually because the fear of pain from a wound makes the patient reluctant to use the abdominal muscles. Encouragement should be given to move the lower limbs and, where allowed, to drink plenty of fluids.

When offered a bed-pan or commode the patient should be given complete privacy. If the patient is allowed to sit out of bed, a commode may prove far more comfortable than a bed-pan and therefore far more effective.

Constipation must be avoided and with good nursing management this can usually be achieved without recourse to laxatives or enemas.

PARALYTIC ILEUS

This is a serious complication in which paralysis and dilatation of the bowel occur. No faeces or flatus can be passed and bowel sounds are absent. Severe abdominal distension and vomiting may occur and the pulse rate is rapid.

A paralytic ileus may be due to extensive handling of the colon during the course of an operation or it may be due to potassium deficiency (p. 42).

Treatment: Oral feeding is stopped and replaced by intravenous fluids. A gastric tube may be passed and fluid aspirated from the stomach or small intestine in an effort to relieve the colon and reduce the abdominal distension. The amount of intravenous fluid given should equal that of the normal intake, plus the amount of fluid aspirated. These amounts must be recorded on the fluid chart.

The patient may become shocked and toxaemic; breathing becomes difficult owing to the abdominal distension and tachycardia is a further sign of distress. Oxygen may be required. Extensive nursing care as for any dangerously ill patient will be needed.

Oral feeding is recommenced when bowel sounds can be heard again through a stethoscope. A further sign of recovery is the passage of flatus per rectum, either normally or by flatus tube.

PULMONARY COMPLICATIONS

These are most common especially following abdominal surgery. They are caused by excessive secretions collecting in the air passages with resultant blockage of the bronchioles. This may occur as a result of:

The inhalation of saliva or vomit whilst unconscious.
The patient lying for a considerable time in one position.
The irritating effect of some anaesthetics and of some pre-operative or post-operative drugs which tend to depress respiration and inhibit the action of the ciliated epithelium lining the major air passages.
Lack of movement and shallow breathing by which the lungs are not fully expanded and the bronchioles remain blocked. This commonly happens where the patient has a wound which makes coughing and deep breathing extremely painful.
Excessive sputum in patients who are heavy smokers or who suffer from bronchitis.

By good nursing and acute observation the number of post-operative chest complications may be reduced considerably. In the first instance the care of the unconscious patient is extremely important, particularly with regard to keeping the airway clear of obstruction following the administration of an anaesthetic (p. 37). Where unconsciousness persists for some time the patient must be turned frequently from side to side and lifted into the upright position as soon as possible after recovery from the anaesthetic, making sure that he is comfortably warm and not in a draught.

Deep breathing and coughing exercises should be commenced as soon as possible. Whilst the patient is attempting to cough the nurse should place her hand firmly but gently over the wound. This gives support, helps to prevent damage to the wound and reassures the patient that coughing can do no harm.

Later the patient should be encouraged to sit forward and place both hands over the wound and cough for about 5 minutes in every hour. Deep breathing should be practised as often as possible. Smoking should be forbidden.

Because they are afraid of causing themselves pain after operation, few patients will breathe deeply without supervision. A simple explanation of the effects of shallow breathing is usually sufficient to gain the co-operation of the patient. Nevertheless, close observation on the respiratory habits of all post-operative patients should be maintained at all times in order to prevent further complications as described below.

Atelectasis (collapse of the lung)

This usually occurs during the second night after operation as a result of a blockage of the bronchioles or as a result of shallow breathing and failure to expand the lungs as described above.

A lung, or part of a lung, collapses into a solid, airless condition, giving rise to respiratory distress of varying degrees. The patient becomes ill with pyrexia and tachycardia. The affected side of the chest becomes flattened, with impaired movement, while movement of the other side is increased.

Treatment Once atelectasis develops, attempts are made to clear the bronchi by exhalations and coughing. Deep breathing and coughing exercises should be carried out for a few minutes in every hour. Care must be taken to ensure that bandages or strapping do not constrict the chest. Where dyspnoea or cyanosis becomes evident, inhalations of oxygen may be ordered.

If the condition of the patient will permit, postural drainage with the bed placed head downwards may dislodge the mucus, allowing the lung to expand. Treatment by the physiotherapist by percussion or tapping of the chest may be carried out. Should all other methods fail, suction or bronchoscopy may be performed by the surgeon.

Pulmonary embolism

This is a blood clot that primarily forms in the veins of the lower leg, usually in the calf, and breaks away from its source of origin, to be carried by the blood stream to the right side of the heart where it blocks the pulmonary artery. If it is large the result is usually fatal, the patient collapsing with little or no warning.

Pulmonary infarct

This is a smaller blood clot that breaks away from a vein as described above and lodges eventually in one of the smaller vessels in the lung. This produces pain in the chest, cough and pyrexia. Later there may be some haemoptysis.

Treatment The patient is often frightened at the symptoms and will need comfort and reassurance. Inhalations of drugs to liquify thick sputum may be administered by passing oxygen through a nebulizer containing the drug. This produces a fine mist to be inhaled by the patient.

Anti-coagulents may be ordered to break down the clot and are usually continued for 3–4 weeks. The anti-coagulent drugs commonly used are *Heparin* and *Dindevan*.

Heparin is given by injection and is used in emergency because it has an immediate action.

Dindevan can be given by mouth and has a lasting action.

THROMBOSIS

This is a condition in which slowing of the venous circulation gives rise to the formation of blood clots in the deep veins. These clots are poorly adherent to the walls of the veins and fragments may separate to be carried in the blood stream to lodge in other parts of the body. The condition arises where patients remain immobile after operation or where undue pressure is placed on the calf muscles.

In order to stimulate the circulation and to prevent thrombosis the patient is got out of bed as soon as possible but in the interim should be persuaded to move the legs about in the bed and to wriggle the toes at frequent intervals. A bed cradle which takes the weight of the bedding from the feet will make this easier to do. Tight bandages must be avoided.

PERITONITIS

This condition is inflammation of the peritoneum as the result of the spread of infection from lesions or perforations in an abdominal organ (p. 82, Fig. 13).

The reaction of the peritoneum gives rise to a copious discharge of fluid. The patient becomes very ill with abdominal pain, pyrexia or hyperpyrexia, rapid pulse rate, varying degrees of dyspnoea, abdominal distension (ascites), nausea and vomiting.

The infection is treated with antibiotics. Morphine and its derivatives may be ordered for the relief of pain and relaxation of the patient. No food is given by mouth and aspiration of the stomach and intestinal contents through a Ryles or gastro-intestinal tube such as a Miller Abbott tube is commenced.

The amount of fluid aspirated must be replaced by intravenous fluids. Antibiotics may be added to the drip through the special rubber section in the delivery tube (p. 47, Fig. 5) after which the infusion should be allowed to run rapidly for a few seconds to ensure that the antibiotic solution does not remain in the vein where it could give rise to venous thrombosis.

The administration of oxygen may become necessary because the abdominal distension makes breathing difficult and the patient may suffer varying degrees of anoxaemia (lack of oxygen in the blood).

A plasma electrolyte estimation is carried out regularly and potassium given as required to prevent or relieve any paralytic ileus that may occur (p. 58).

The patient is nursed in the upright position and on complete bed rest. All pressure points must be watched carefully because, owing to the acute pain and abdominal distension, movement is very difficult for the patient and the skin rapidly becomes sore.

The maintenance of oral hygiene is most important: frequent mouth washes should be given.

PARESIS

This is partial paralysis, often of an arm. This may be caused by pressure on the nerves, e.g. the brachial plexus at the side of the neck and under the clavicle or the radial nerve at the back of the arm, following a prolonged operation. It may also arise from over-abduction of the arm in the 'drip position'.

Paresis can occur as the result of injury to the nerves when a limb of an unconscious patient is allowed to hang over the side of a bed or of a trolley during transit from the theatre to the ward. This is the result of carelessness on the part of those in charge of the patient and one which no good nurse would allow.

Any post-operative weakness or loss of movement of a limb must be reported immediately so that physiotherapy may be started without delay.

WOUND RUPTURE

Occasionally a wound will break down and rupture from 7 to 10 days after operation. Several factors may be responsible for disruption of a wound and may include faulty catgut used in closing the wound in the theatre, strain on the wound from excessive vomiting or coughing, anaemia, delayed healing due to the poor general condition of the patient, blood collecting in the wound (haematoma) or infection.

If a dressing which should be dry is unusually wet, or if a patient complains that all is not well with the wound, disruption of a wound may be suspected. The wound must not be touched or inspected until a sterile dressing trolley is ready at the bedside. If the rupture is found to be severe, the wound is covered with moist saline packs of gauze (not cotton wool) and a firm many-tailed bandage applied. The doctor must be notified and arrangements made for the patient to return to the theatre for re-suturing. The patient's confidence will be undermined by such an occurrence and will need a great deal of calm reassurance..

HAEMATOMA

This is a blood clot in the wound giving rise to pain and bulging of the wound and breakdown of the edges. Where the clot is not too large a suture may be removed and the clot expressed but if the haematoma is extensive a return to the theatre may be necessary to evacuate the collected blood and re-suture the wound. A haematoma in a wound may cause infection.

INFECTION

Infection may enter a wound from equipment that is inefficiently sterilized, by careless handling of sterilized equipment or faulty dressing techniques.

Dressings covering clean wounds are normally handled as little as possible and then only by the 'non-touch' technique (p. 75).

The wound should be inspected if the patient complains of unusual pain, if there is excessive exudation from the wound and if there is a rise in temperature.

FISTULA

A fistula is an abnormal channel leading from an internal organ to the skin surface or from the cavity of one organ to another, e.g. a fistula leading from the bladder through into the rectum (*retrovesical fistula*) or a *faecal fistula* from the intestine to the surface.

An abdominal fistula may deliberately be made by the surgeon for drainage purposes as in cholecystotomy (drainage of the gall bladder). The deliberate fistula may be a temporary measure, in which case it is closed by surgery when it has served its purpose, or it may be permanent. A colostomy following excision of the rectum is an example of a permanent fistula.

A faecal fistula may follow operation for the removal of a gangrenous appendix. Other faecal fistulae may develop after resection of any part of the colon. In such cases copious discharge is poured out over the surface of the wound. Great care must be taken to ensure that the skin around the external opening of the fistula is prevented from becoming sore. Frequent application of a barrier cream should be made to protect the skin. Skilful nursing will be necessary.

SINUS

Occasionally a deep wound will heal almost completely except for a tract leading from the surface of the wound to the underlying tissues. The walls of a sinus are lined with granulation tissue which is slow to heal and continues discharging in spite of treatment. (Granulation tissue must be swabbed very carefully when doing a dressing or it may bleed profusely or be destroyed.) Occasionally a sinus may be due to a tiny piece of ligature in the tissues and will persist until it is removed.

SURGICAL EMPHYSEMA

This condition is the presence of air in the subcutaneous tissues causing swelling. Crackling sounds (crepitus) are heard when the skin is touched. It is most often seen as a complication of fractured ribs when the pleura is punctured or following a punctured wound (p. 5) where air may be drawn into the tissues. Air may also be introduced through an infected wound as in gas gangrene (p. 24).

Surgical emphysema is not common and may be overlooked in its first stages. The slightest swelling accompanied by the feel or sound of crackling under the skin must be reported without delay. The condition usually subsides within a few days but during that time the patient suffers distress and discomfort from the tightness of the skin and the rather frightening sensation of air in the tissues. Very often the swelling closes the eyes which adds to the discomfort.

Where the emphysema affects any part of the trunk or limbs, frequent attention must be given to the pressure areas because the skin under such pressure is likely to split within a very short time.

BEDSORES

These occur chiefly in chronically ill or debilitated patients suffering from protein deficiency or malnutrition, in obese or very thin patients, or in unconscious or otherwise helpless patients. They may be the result of the poor general condition of the patient, pressure or friction from the bed, splints or other apparatus or from moisture in the bed. These predisposing conditions can be alleviated with good nursing and, except in rare instances, the nurses in charge of a patient are responsible if a bedsore develops.

Bedsores can develop into ulcers in a very few hours, usually without the knowledge of the patient because the lesions are relatively painless. Herein lies the danger of an impending bedsore and the importance of constant supervision and preventive treatment.

In the prevention of bedsores in the surgical ward the particular circumstances and condition of each patient must be taken into account. Following a prolonged operation, in which the patient has remained in one position on the operating table, the skin must be carefully examined for any signs of reddening (erythema) or bruising as soon as possible after the return to the ward and treated accordingly. Whilst unconscious the position of the patient should be changed frequently. Patients having a painful wound will be reluctant to move about in the bed and should be assisted and encouraged to move as much as possible.

Wrist watches and rings, other than wedding rings, should never be worn by nurses when carrying out nursing procedures because these can tear or scratch the patient's skin and bedsores may result. Severely ill and helpless patients should be lifted clear of the bed by *two* nurses when giving and removing bed-pans. When draw sheets are changed they should be rolled into place and never pulled from underneath a patient. The skin covering the buttocks and sacral area is easily damaged by careless handling.

If the skin is broken or a bedsore has developed, the lesion, however small, must be treated as any other open wound. Sterile dressings used under strict aseptic precautions become essential. Where conditions are suitable the doctor may allow the patient with an impending bedsore to sit out of bed in order to relieve pressure on the affected part of the body, but it must be remembered that sitting in a chair for any length of time also entails pressure on some part of the body. Air rings or cushions must be provided and the patient well supported and made really comfortable with pillows and, if possible, a footstool.

All threatened bedsores, without exception, must be reported without delay so that treatment may be started immediately.

PLASTER SORES

Plaster of paris casts may be applied following orthopaedic operations on bones or joints or the reduction of a fracture.

Swelling occurring beneath a plaster cast cannot be foreseen by the surgeon in the theatre and the greatest danger is that the plaster may become too tight with resultant interference with the venous circulation of the limb. If neglected, this in turn will lead to gangrene and the possible loss of a limb.

When a plaster splint is applied the fingers and toes are always left exposed so that they may be watched by day and night for any signs of undue pressure causing constriction of the blood vessels. Discoloration of the skin and nails, coldness, loss of feeling or movement, must be reported immediately. Every complaint, however trivial, made by a patient in plaster must be investigated. Pain under the edges of the plaster may indicate increased pressure on the limb and must be relieved as soon as possible. The insertion of pieces of cotton wool is useless and dangerous because the wool becomes hard and tends only to increase further the pressure. The matter must be reported and the surgeon will decide on the course of action to be taken.

Pressure sores or ulcers may occur also *inside* a plaster cast, the signs and symptoms being pyrexia, restlessness, pain and sleeplessness. In extreme cases an offensive odour and staining of the plaster by discharge will indicate the presence of suppuration beneath the plaster; an occurrence we hope never to see in the hospital ward.

Trimming the edges of, or cutting windows in, the plaster splints to relieve pressure or friction is entirely the province of the medical staff and must not be attempted by a nurse; but it is the nurse who, by her observation and care, can do so much to avoid severe damage to, or even the loss of, a limb.

GENERAL OBSERVATIONS

After operation the condition of the majority of patients progresses to a satisfactory conclusion but there is an ever-present danger that unforeseen complications may arise.

Once the patient has left the theatre, the surgeons rely on the nursing staff for close observation of the patient and information regarding progress because the nurse is in constant contact with the patient and is in the position to notice and to report any deviation from normal recovery.

After studying the incidence of post-operative complications, it will be seen that the most preventable can usually be attributed to post-operative immobilization of the patient and failure to breathe efficiently but there are many other signs and symptoms that the surgical nurse must watch for and be able to recognize. Some of these will be obvious only to the nurse; others may be brought to her attention in complaints from the patients themselves, and in regard to this, the nurse should be particularly careful and alert with the apparently fussy, oft-complaining patient, because at some time one of the complaints made by such a patient may be a genuine sign of the onset of a post-operative complication. Pain is nature's way of warning the body and no pain should be ignored, especially where it is continuous or appears to be remote from the site of the operation.

The slightest lapse from the normal in the condition of a patient must be reported to senior nursing staff or to the doctor without delay. Where abnormal signs or symptoms become evident, the nurse should show no signs of anxiety or concern but should proceed in a calm and confident manner. Even where swift and positive action becomes imperative, speed can be achieved without fuss: the sight of a nurse *running* through the ward can cause feelings of panic in other patients.

Most patients become anxious when they realize that complications have arisen and, spoken or unspoken, the question will be 'what is going to happen to me?' Every effort must be made to reassure and restore confidence in the patient.

13. DISINFECTION AND STERILIZATION

Certain terms are used to describe means of preventing the growth of and the destruction of micro-organisms and their spores.

Asepsis means freedom from micro-organisms and their spores.

Antisepsis is the use of chemical substances that check the growth of micro-organisms but do not destroy them.

Sepsis is the infection of the body by pyogenic organisms.

Disinfection implies the use of liquid agents that will kill bacteria but *not their spores.* Bacteria readily grow in watery solutions and many disinfectants diluted in water become a source of danger. After a short time the disinfectant deteriorates and becomes ineffective enabling micro-organisms to live and multiply in the solution. Where disinfectants are used in the ward, fresh supplies should be prepared each day and the remains of old solutions thrown away, otherwise it is never certain that all bacteria are destroyed. Micro-organisms do not survive in alcoholic solutions, therefore spirit is most useful in disinfecting sharp instruments. Articles to be disinfected must be completely covered by the solution.

Sterilization is the process whereby the aseptic condition of equipment is ensured, commonly by the application of extreme heat in various forms as follows:

(i) Dry heat such as baking in ovens through which hot air is circulated: a method often used in the sterilization of syringes and needles.

(ii) Moist heat: (a) Boiling, by which the articles to be sterilized are completely immersed in water and boiled for at least five

minutes *timed from the moment the water boils* and not before. Each time an article is placed in the sterilizer the rest of the contents must be considered to be unsterile for a further five minutes. This method is commonly used for the ward sterilization of non-disposable blunt instruments, enamel ware and rubber or metal equipment but is considered to be unsatisfactory in that boiling will kill micro-organisms but does not destroy spores.

(b) Steam under pressure or autoclaving. Articles to be sterilized are subjected to steam under pressure for a specified time then thoroughly dried by vacuum. Dressings, dressing towels, surgical caps and gowns, etc., are packed loosely into perforated drums or boxes which enable the steam to penetrate their contents. Surgical gloves should be packed into special glove boxes and autoclaved separately at a lower temperature because a lower steam pressure is required for rubber or latex equipment. The perforations in the dressing drums or boxes are closed immediately they are taken from the autoclave. If the contents are found to be damp on opening the drum, this means that they are not sterile and must not be used. The drum should be repacked and returned for re-sterilization.

Ward sterilization of non-disposable equipment

Every article must be thoroughly cleaned and inspected for stains or debris before being sterilized. *Enamel* ware is washed in hot, soapy water and rinsed. *Blunt* instruments should be scrubbed with a stiff brush to ensure that all crevices and grooves are immaculately clean. Instruments with *grooved* ends such as artery forceps, sinus forceps and sponge holders, etc., should be placed in the sterilizer in the open position so that every tiny crevice is exposed to the sterilizing agent. The addition of sodium bicarbonate to the water reduces the risk of rust on metal instruments.

Sharp instruments should not be boiled as this blunts the sharp edges of scissors, scalpels and needles. They should be thoroughly cleaned and dried then immersed in a disinfectant such as Dettol in spirit, Hibitane 1–250 or the disinfectant currently in use in the ward.

Glass is easily broken when boiled. It should be wrapped in old lint or cotton material, placed in cool water and brought to the boil.

Rubber may also be sterilized by boiling but will deteriorate eventually with frequent boiling.

CENTRAL STERILIZATION SUPPLY DEPARTMENT

An increasing number of hospitals are now using pre-sterilized equipment prepared in a Central Sterilizing Supply Department (C.S.S.D.). Here everything needed for any aseptic procedure anywhere in the hospital is packed by non-nursing staff into individual packs. These are double wrapped with an outer covering of a special type of paper that can be penetrated by the sterilizing agent. To each pack is attached a sensitive strip that changes colour when sterilization is complete. All packs and boxes must be carefully checked by the nurse before use. The contents will be unsterile where the control strip has not changed colour or where any part of the outer covering is punctured or otherwise damaged. Such defective packs must be returned for re-sterilizing.

From the C.S.S.D. these individual packs are distributed to the wards and departments of the hospital daily, as required.

Bowls, trays, gallipots, syringes and many instruments are now manufactured from plastic materials or aluminium foil that can be thrown away after use. All types of towels, including dressing towels, are made of toughened paper and paper bags are supplied as receivers for soiled dressings and instruments. Special packs can be assembled to contain anything that may be needed.

Non-disposable instruments are returned to the C.S.S.D. after use for cleaning, sterilizing and re-packing. In some hospitals special pre-set trays are prepared and sterilized in the C.S.S.D. for use in the theatre for individual operations.

Sterilization of equipment in the C.S.S.D. is carried out by means of gamma radiation or by autoclaving.

14. WARD DRESSINGS

GENERAL PRECAUTIONS

In surgical nursing the aim is to keep sterile wounds free from infection and to assist healing. To achieve this it is necessary for the nurse to be constantly aware of what is taking place in the ward in relation to the surgical care of the patient. Methods of carrying out dressings and other sterile procedures may vary in minor detail from hospital to hospital and sometimes from one ward to another according to the wishes of the surgeons or of the senior nursing staff, but the basic principles remain constant.

No sterile trolleys should be prepared or wounds exposed as long as there is any dust-raising activity taking place in the ward such as sweeping, dusting or bed-making.

A surgery adjacent to the ward, into which the beds can be wheeled and dressings can be changed, is an ideal arrangement, but where this is not possible, the greatest care must be taken when renewing or inspecting each dressing in the ward.

Clean wounds must be dressed first; septic wounds last.

A clean wound is usually left untouched until the stitches or clips are to be removed. Where a patient having a clean wound complains of pain, swelling or inflammation, or if pyrexia or a rapid pulse intervenes, the wound must be inspected because these are signs of possible infection. When such inspection becomes necessary, a corner of a dressing must NEVER be lifted to 'take a peep'. This is most dangerous because, apart from being contaminated by the fingers, the dressing is invariably shifted, allowing micro-organisms access into the wound with risk of further infection. A sterile trolley must be prepared and the wound inspected under full aseptic conditions.

To avoid raising dust and fluff when preparing a patient, the screens should be pulled gently and the bedding disturbed as little as possible and, to reduce the risk of droplet infection, talking between nurses and/or the patient should be reduced to a minimum whilst dressing a wound. A wound must not be exposed until the sterile trolley is at the bedside and everything is ready for the renewal of the dressing.

Hands cannot be made sterile but by careful and thorough washing, rinsing and drying, superficial bacteria may be removed from the skin. Where possible, paper towels should be used for drying the hands. Drying the hands and arms prevents drips of unsterile water from falling on the sterile field, on the trolley or on to the wound. A fresh towel should be used and discarded between each dressing. Care must be taken to ensure that the hands touch nothing on the way from the sink to the patient's bedside.

When the last dressing is completed and the trolley cleared, the nurse should again wash her hands and apply hand cream or lotion to keep the skin soft and in good condition and to prevent chafing of the hands especially in cold weather.

Where disposable face masks are worn, a fresh one should be worn for each dressing. Whilst carrying out any sterile procedure the mask should not be touched by the fingers nor allowed to hang round the neck. On completion of each dressing masks should be thrown away. They should never be put into uniform pockets.

BASIC WARD DRESSING PROCEDURE

Immediately before starting a dressing the trolley shelves and rails should be cleaned with soapy water, rinsed and dried with a disposable towel which must then be discarded.

All unsterile equipment is placed on the lower shelf including lotions, adhesive plaster, bandages, dressing packs and instrument packs as required. The top shelf is left clear for sterile articles only (Fig. 8). Where pre-sterilized packs are not available, bowls and instruments should not be removed from the sterilizer until the last moment and should be covered with a sterile towel whilst the trolley is being taken to the bedside.

Basic dressing packs from the C.S.S.D. contain approximately 5 wool swabs, gauze swabs, 2 plastic or foil gallipots, one or two dressing towels, 2 pairs of dressing forceps and a pair of surgical scissors. The contents of a standard dressing pack may vary slightly in different hospitals but the basic equipment is fundamentally the same. Extra instruments that may be required are supplied in separate cylindrical packs.

When opening a dressing pack the sealing tape is cut cleanly across its width with scissors that are kept in spirit and used solely for this purpose. Fragments from the outer envelope

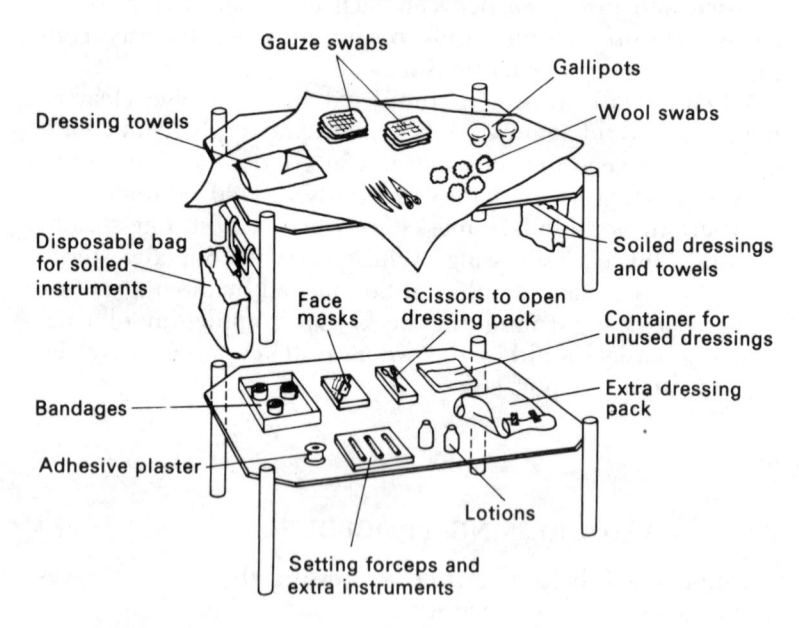

Fig. 8. Basic dressing trolley

must not be allowed to fall on to the top of the trolley. Great care must be taken that the fingers do not come into contact with the upper edges of the outer covering of the pack or the sterile contents will become contaminated as it is being extracted. In some hospitals sterile forceps taken from a pre-sterilized cylinder (Fig. 9) are used to remove the inner sterile pack and again extreme care must be taken to ensure that neither the forceps nor the sterile pack come into contact with any part of the outer envelope. In other hospitals the inner pack is tipped out on to the top shelf of the trolley. Where this method is adopted the outer pack must be so held that the sterile pack falls on to the trolley with the free edges uppermost allowing direct access to the contents. When unfolded, the wrapper becomes a sterile towel on which to arrange the equipment needed for the dressing.

The bed is screened and the bedding and the patient's clothing so arranged that only the area of the wound is exposed. This should be done quietly and smoothly and the patient made as comfortable as possible. Meanwhile the nurse should take the opportunity of explaining the procedure to the

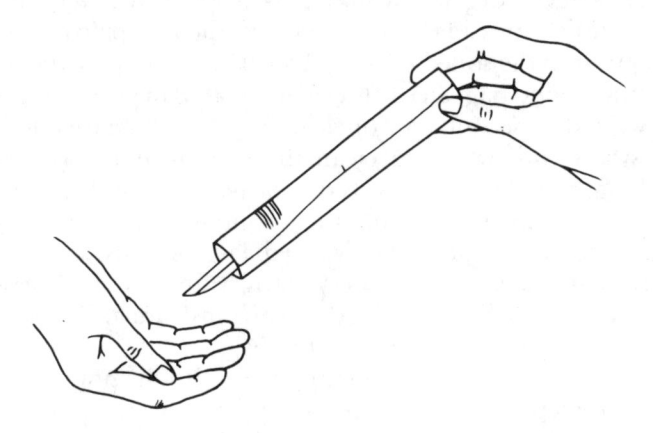

Fig. 9. Pre-sterilized instrument tipped directly into dresser's hand

patient who, if it is a first dressing after operation, may understandably be feeling apprehensive if not actually frightened.

The bandage or adhesive plaster holding the dressing in place is removed by the dresser's assistant but the dressing itself is left intact until all the preliminary preparations for its renewal are completed.

The non-touch technique is adopted for all dressings. This means that neither the dressings covering a wound nor the wound itself are touched with bare hands. Sterile forceps are always used as a second pair of hands thus safeguarding both nurse and patient from any risk of cross infection.

The assistant dresser opens the dressing pack as described above, the inner pack is placed in readiness on the trolley shelf.

The bag forming the outer covering of the pack is fastened to the trolley rail with adhesive strapping to serve as a disposable receptacle for soiled dressings. A second bag is attached to the opposite rail into which instruments are placed after use.

The dresser washes and dries her hands and, using a pair of sterile forceps, opens out the aseptic dressing pack and arranges the swabs, instruments and gallipots. The assistant pours the required lotions into the gallipots. (Care must be taken that no drips fall on to the paper towel covering the trolley—micro-organisms may pass through the wet patch.)

The soiled dressing is removed with the first pair of forceps and put into the soiled dressing bag. The forceps are discarded into the second bag. Sterile towels are placed in position around the wound. A second pair of clean forceps is then used to hold the swabs with which to clean the area around the wound, working *away* from the incision to avoid the risk of micro-organisms being washed into the wound from the surrounding skin. The wound itself is cleansed last. At this stage other instruments such as sinus forceps, artery forceps, stitch scissors or a probe may be needed. After each instrument is used it is placed into the correct disposable bag.

Finally, the clean dressing is applied with still another pair of sterile forceps. The bandage is replaced or re-applied, the pillows and bedding rearranged and the patient left comfortable.

On clearing the trolley, every disposable bag must be closed firmly by twisting the opening. Non-disposable articles are returned to the C.S.S.D. for cleaning, sorting and re-sterilizing. Dregs of antiseptics must be thrown away and the trolley relaid for the next dressing.

WOUND DRAINAGE

Where there is likely to be discharge of any kind from a wound, such as pus, blood, serum, urine or bile, a drainage tube is inserted into the wound by the surgeon to afford an open channel for drainage. Drains are made of pieces of fine sheet rubber, corrugated rubber or tubing with or without holes. Ribbon gauze may also be used but this usually requires to be changed daily.

Some drains are secured by a suture or are prevented from slipping back into the wound by a large sterile safety pin inserted at the uppermost end of the tube. When a tube is shortened the end is snipped off and the safety pin replaced by another.

The skin surrounding a drainage tube needs to be protected, with a barrier cream, from any exudate that may cause soreness and chafing.

The intervals of shortening or removing a drainage tube are determined by the surgeon and no action must be taken by nurses until written instructions on this are received from the medical staff.

WOUND COVERINGS

The types of dressings and the method of covering wounds may vary considerably, mainly according to the preference of the surgeon and to the nature of the wound.

The use of pads of cotton wool to cover a wound is becoming obsolete, many surgeons preferring plastic skin dressings such as *Nobecutane* or *Octaflex* which are sprayed over the incision to provide a transparent film adherent to the skin, making bandages unnecessary.

The 'window' dressing is another advance in wound covering where sterilized celophane is placed over a wound and secured to the skin by adhesive tape on all sides of the 'window'.

Moist wounds, or those having excessive and persistent exudation with or without drainage tubes, do need a covering of absorbent cotton wool and, in some cases, an outer layer of non-absorbent wool is necessary to avoid soiling of bandages or bedding.

REMOVAL OF CLIPS AND STITCHES

A sterile trolley must be prepared for the removal of clips and stitches. The incision must be kept *dry*. Swabbing with

78 FOUNDATIONS OF SURGICAL NURSING

antiseptics either before or after removal of the sutures or clips may be the means of introducing micro-organisms into the tiny punctures left on the skin.

Michel's clips are small metal strips with a tiny tooth of metal at each end. Michel's forceps are used to remove the clips. The curved blade is placed under the central portion of the strip and the forceps closed. The ends of the Michel's clips rise clear of the skin (Fig. 10a).

Kifa clips are removed by squeezing together the two wings on the upper surface of the clips with forceps (Fig. 10b).

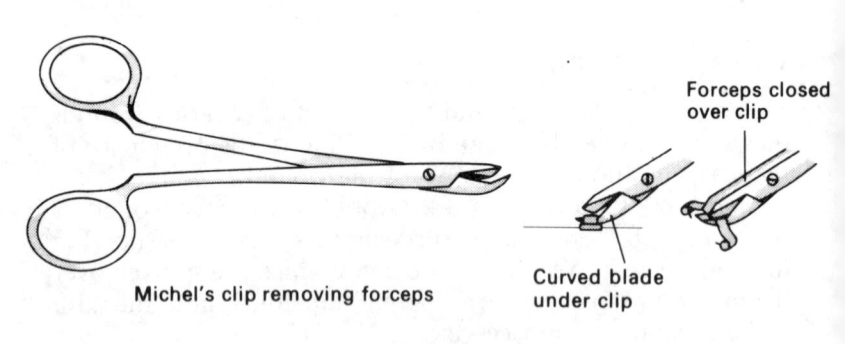

Michel's clip removing forceps

Curved blade under clip

Forceps closed over clip

(a) *Removal of Michel's clips*

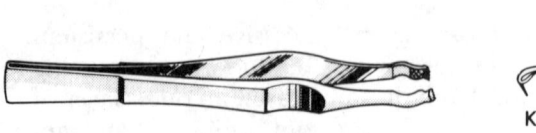

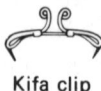

Kifa clip

Wings of Kifa c pressed togeth with forceps fo removal

(b) *Method of removing Kifa clips*

Stitches

To remove stitches the blades of the scissors or of the stitch cutter must be held parallel to the skin to avoid pricking or scratching. The knot of the suture is held with forceps and raised sufficiently to allow the point of the scissors to be inserted. The stitch is cut between the knot and the skin. With the knot held firmly in the forceps, the stitch is drawn out (Fig. 11).

Following the removal of clips or stitches, the wound may be left dry and uncovered or, in certain cases, a spray dressing may be applied.

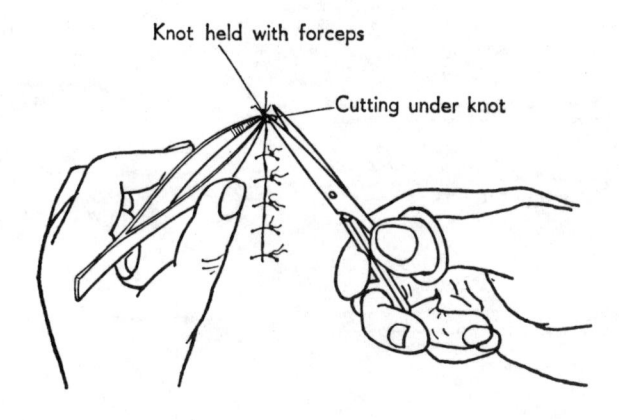

Fig. 11. Removal of stitches

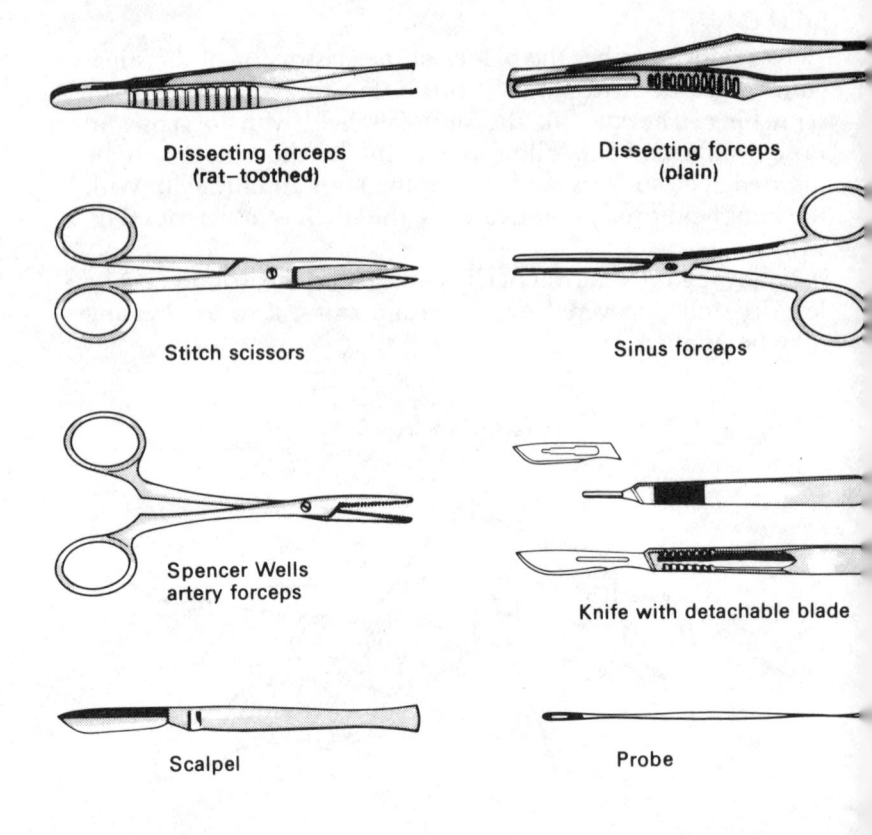

Fig. 12. Surgical instruments

15. SURGICAL EMERGENCIES

Emergency operations are those performed as soon as possible after admission in order to save life. Apart from accidental injuries, surgical emergencies are mainly concerned with some obstruction or perforation of the internal organs of the body, chiefly in the abdominal cavity (Fig. 13).

For the sake of convenience in describing various parts of the abdomen, it is figuratively divided into anatomical areas (Fig. 14). Special terms are used to denote each of these areas which a doctor invariably uses when entering the history and diagnosis on the patient's case sheet.

As very little is known about the condition of the patient in an emergency admission, it is essential that before arrival in the ward, all equipment needed for use in such emergencies as haemorrhage, shock or excessive vomiting should be placed near the bed, so that it is readily accessible. This should include oxygen and suction apparatus, bed elevators, drip stand, a tray containing a vomit bowl and paper towels on the locker and an examination tray in readiness for the medical staff.

On admission the patient is made comfortable and the doctor notified. If shock or haemorrhage are evident these must be treated without delay. Any degree of shock must be overcome before the administration of anaesthesia otherwise the condition may be aggravated by the operation, resulting in the collapse and death of the patient. Nothing should be given by mouth until the patient has been examined by the surgeon and the diagnosis is confirmed. A mouth wash may be allowed but must not be swallowed.

Where the condition of the patient permits the nurse should endeavour to obtain the following information:

(a) How long before admission the last food or drink was taken (this has an important bearing on the administration of anaesthetic and the risk of vomiting during operation).

(b) Whether the patient is a cigarette smoker and, if so, how many per day are consumed.

(c) If the patient has taken any drugs, even aspirin, prior to admission. This is doubly important if insulin, steroids or anticoagulents are being taken as routine treatment. Patients on these drugs are issued with a card stating the name of the drug, the dosage and the time it should be taken. This card should be carried on the person at all times but in a surgical emergency it may have been forgotten by the patient. The nurse must then try to obtain the required information and to make a note of it.

The nurse should note whether any physical abnormalities are evident or if the patient shows signs of abnormal behaviour.

Following examination by the doctor, special investigations will be made with no loss of time and may include x-rays, blood and urine tests and the collection of various specimens for laboratory examination and reports.

Where the general condition of the patient is unsatisfactory,

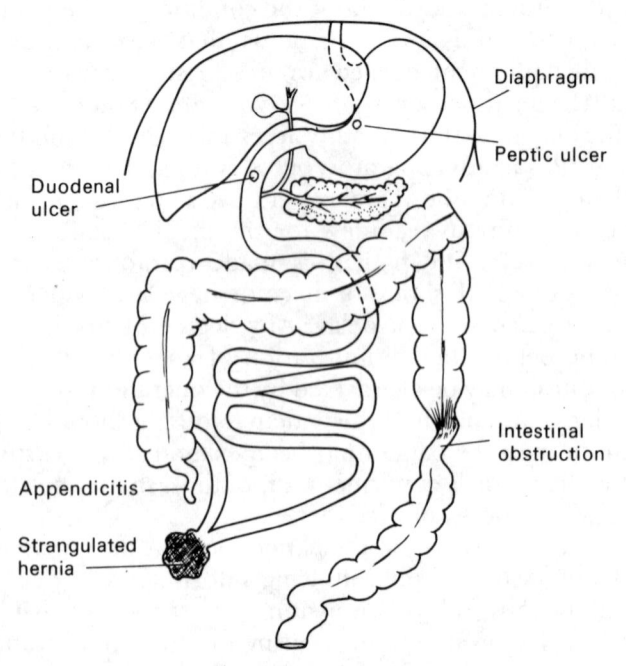

Fig. 13. Sites of common surgical emergencies

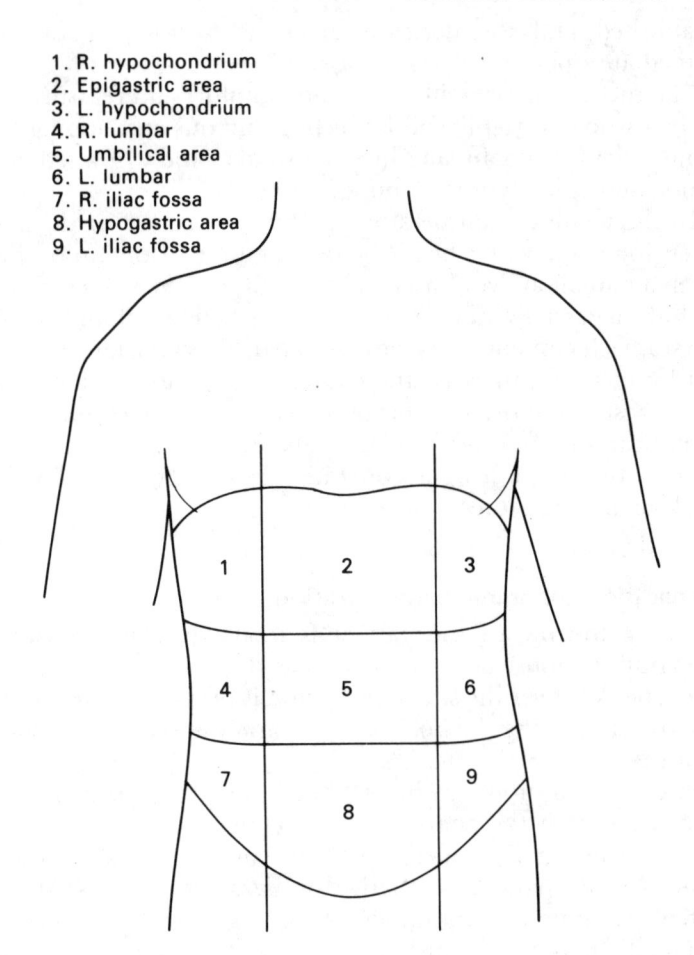

1. R. hypochondrium
2. Epigastric area
3. L. hypochondrium
4. R. lumbar
5. Umbilical area
6. L. lumbar
7. R. iliac fossa
8. Hypogastric area
9. L. iliac fossa

Fig. 14. Abdominal areas

every effort is made to bring about an improvement so that the patient will be better able to withstand the effects of an operation. Special treatment may be required for those suffering from diseases or defects of the heart or lungs, from diabetes or dehydration, etc.

Very often a patient admitted for an emergency operation is suffering pain and will invariably ask for sedatives. Drugs for the relief of pain are not given until the doctor has seen the patient, diagnosis is confirmed, the site and extent of pain established and the decision made as to whether or not immediate operation is essential.

The nurse will need all her skill to comfort and reassure the patient who invariably will be feeling anxious and hoping for rapid relief from pain, and may not understand why a sedative is not immediately forthcoming.

In the routine pre-operative treatment no food or drink is given for from 4 to 5 hours before the time of operation but when a patient arrives for emergency surgery the stomach may be full or partially full. Before an anaesthetic is administered, the stomach contents must be evacuated. This is usually carried out by suction, otherwise the patient is likely to vomit during anaesthesia, a most dangerous occurrence that could cause complications if vomitus is inhaled into the lungs, added to which, vomiting during an operation may seriously delay the work of the surgeon.

Preparation for immediate operation

Where the life of the patient is in danger, pre-operative preparations must be carried out swiftly.

1. The skin over the site of operation is prepared in the usual way (p. 31), leaving the final skin preparation to be done in the theatre.

2. Catheterization may be ordered if the patient is unable to pass urine or if the abdomen is distended.

3. Watches and jewellery must be removed and signed for, either by the patient, a relative or by a senior nurse if the patient is alone and incapable of signing.

4. All make-up must be removed because artificial colouring, especially on the finger nails, masks any evidence of cyanosis, making it difficult for the anaesthetist to judge the condition during and immediately following anaesthesia.

5. Dentures are removed and placed in antiseptic and put in a safe place.

6. An identification band must be fastened round the wrist or ankle. The name on the band must be *exactly* the same as that on the patient's case sheet and must be checked before the patient leaves the ward for the operating theatre (p. 32).

7. Where a life is in danger, pre-medication is often given intravenously for a rapid result.

8. The patient should not be left alone and no comment whatsoever regarding the condition, diagnosis or impending operation should be made by a nurse within hearing of the patient or to relatives or others accompanying the patient. All enquiries must be referred to the senior nurse in charge of the ward or to the doctor. Normally the consent for operation is signed either by the patient or by a relative but where the patient is admitted alone and is incapable of signing, the matter is left to the discretion of the surgeon who will decide on the course of action according to the condition of the patient and the danger of loss of life.

16. CARE OF THE ELDERLY

With increasing age various physical and mental disorders arise that in many instances have some bearing on the pre-operative and post-operative treatment and recovery. These ailments are usually of long-standing duration and include *osteo-arthritis* and *rheumatoid arthritis* that render movement both difficult and very painful, facts that must be remembered when moving the patient.

Diseases of the *upper respiratory tract*, such as bronchitis, that give rise to bouts of coughing and dyspnoea are commonly found in the elderly patient and may cause severe post-operative pulmonary complications (p. 59).

Diseases of the *heart* and *circulatory system* are also common in the elderly, the patient showing signs of respiratory distress, cyanosis and, in severe cases, threatened gangrene of the extremities due to impaired circulation. Also the walls of the veins lose their elasticity and more easily tend to become varicosed, with resulting stagnation of blood in the veins. Herein lies the danger of post-operative thrombosis or embolism (p. 61).

Gentle movement of the limbs in pre-operative and post-operative treatment is important but manual assistance from the nurse will be needed for this because the muscular exertion required may be a physical hazard for a patient with a cardio-vascular disability.

Urinary disorders in the elderly mainly arise because of loss of muscle tone. The muscle walls and sphincters of the bladder become weak and difficult to control with the result that frequency and incontinence of urine intervene.

In many cases these symptoms are aggravated by feelings of anxiety or stress, apart from the pain the patient may be suffering or the thought of an impending operation.

Most aged patients become very distressed not only at being

removed from their homes, whatever the reason, but also with the lack of privacy, the loss of independence and, too often, the regrettable familiarity with which they are addressed by some hospital staff, nurses included. An unmarried lady or gentleman does not appreciate being called 'granny' or 'granddad' or indeed by any other appellation other than their own, whatever their status in life. Such discourtesy is often silently resented, causing stress and irritation which a patient may endeavour to suppress but which may be resolved in some physical disorder of which frequency or incontinence may be an example.

Pressure sores are a real danger, both in pre-operative and post-operative nursing as described on p. 65. As soon as the physical condition permits, elderly patients are helped out of bed into a chair. This is beneficial in that it entails movement of the whole body with increased circulation. Nevertheless, sitting in a chair does not prevent pressure sores; the same amount of pressure is put upon the sacral area and the patient is inclined to sit very still in one position.

Care must be taken in ensuring that an aged patient is sitting comfortably, preferably on a soft pillow or cushion, with the back and head well supported with pillows. The back should be as straight as is conducive to comfort so that no pressure or strain is felt on a wound. When in the sitting position there should be no pressure from the edge of the seat on the back of the legs, either above or below the knees. Such pressure may cause the blood to clot in the veins. If a footstool is used the knees should be slightly bent for maximum comfort and relaxation.

It is extremely important that the patient should not be left sitting in a chair for too long a period and on return to bed the pressure areas must be examined for any signs of redness or chafing of the skin.

Undernourishment and **dehydration** are factors that need to be corrected, before operation where possible. Some elderly people are not in the habit of eating or drinking a great deal, either for social reasons where the supply and preparation of food becomes too difficult for them to manage, for financial reasons where food is too expensive or simply because they are too ill or too tired to make the effort to prepare a meal. Such conditions exist where an aged person lives alone. Over a period of time, insufficient nourishment with the associated lack of vitamins, fluids and electrolytes, combined with the physical changes that arise with advancing age, does mean that an elderly person often has less resistance and cannot withstand the effects of a surgical operation as successfully as does a younger person.

Good nutrition is vital in ensuring the restoration and maintenance of health tissue and the successful healing of a wound. The fluid intake must be adequate but not excessive. Many elderly patients cannot take large quantities of food; small portions should be served as attractively as possible and the patient encouraged to eat. A second helping can always be offered and may appeal to the patient far more than one large helping.

Post-operatively the correct balance of fluids and electrolytes is important, particularly the potassium and sodium intake. Inevitably all patients lose fluid during operation but in elderly people, who may be somewhat dehydrated on admission, the replacement of fluid may be essential to recovery and survival. Where intravenous infusions are given they are administered slowly to avoid any degree of oedema caused by fluid collecting in the tissues.

During the days following operation a state of general exhaustion may become evident. The blood pressure must be watched for any signs of impending shock. Any fall in the blood pressure must be reported without delay (p. 39).

The elderly or aged patient often faces operation with somewhat more equanimity than a younger patient may do and often requires less sedation but occasionally the effect of some drugs that may have been given either before or after operation may tend to induce post-operative changes in the mental state leading to confusion when the patient may attempt to get out of bed unaided. Even minor changes in behaviour must be noted and reported but the nurse must be very sure that the apparent confusion is not the result of misunderstanding due to any degree of deafness. The greatest danger in this context is from a patient who is only partially deaf and, finding it difficult to understand what is required, may become irritable or fractious.

Where a confused state *is* established, cot sides or bed rails must be attached to the bed for the safety of the patient. An elderly patient falling out of bed is a serious occurrence from which collapse or death may ensue.

A SHORT LIST OF SURGICAL AND ALLIED TERMS

ANASTAMOSIS   The surgical union of two hollow structures, e.g. gastro-jejunostomy.
ECTOMY (EXCISION)   To cut away, e.g. excision of colon or tumour.
INCISE   To cut into, e.g. incision of an abscess.
LIGATE   To tie, e.g. ligation of blood vessels during operation.
LUMEN   Space inside a tube.
OMA   A tumour of.
OSCOPY   Visual examination of the interior of an organ, e.g. cystoscopy (examination of the bladder).
OSTOMY   Formation of a new opening to the skin surface, e.g. colostomy.
OTOMY   A temporary opening into an organ.
PLASTY   Reconstruction, e.g. arthroplasty of a joint.
STENOSIS   Narrowing of a canal or lumen as in pyloric stenosis of the stomach.

Anatomical prefixes

TRACH	Trachea	CYST	Bladder
BRONCH	Bronchus	PROCT	Rectum
CHOLE	Gall bladder	MAST	Breast
ENTRO	Small intestine	HYSTER	Uterus
HEPAT	Liver	THROMB	Blood clot
PYELO	Pelvis of kidney	PHLEB	Vein
NEPHR	Kidney		

INDEX

Abdomen, areas of, 81
Abrasions, 4
Abscess, stitch, 14
Adherent scars, 7
Admission of, patients, 2
   surgical emergencies, 49
Aerobic bacteria, 16
Aminosol, 51
Anaerobic bacteria, 16
Anaesthetics, 34
Analgesia, 34
Anions, 42
Anoxia, 23
Antibiotics, 28
Anti-coagulent drugs, 61
Anti-diuretic hormone, 42
Antisepsis, 69
Anuria, 57
Asepsis, 69
Aspiration of stomach, 40
Atalectasis, 60
Autoclaving, 70

Bacteria, 16
Bard-Parker blade, 50
Basic dressing pack, 73
Bedding, 20
Bedsores, 65
Blood,
   cross matching, 45
   grouping, 45
   pressure, 39
   transfusion, 45

Carbachol, 57
Casualty department, 6
Catheterization, 57
Cations, 42
Cellulitis, 25
Chemotherapy, 28
Chlorpromazine, 56
Cholecystotomy, 64
Clostridium welchi, 24
   sporoganes, 24
Colostomy, 64
Condylomata, 27
Congenital syphilis, 27
Consent form, 3

Constipation, 58
Contraction of tissues, 8
Contusions, 4
Crepitus, 65
Cross infection, 18
C.S.S.D., 71
Cyanosis, 37
Cyclizine, 56

Dehydration, 87
Dextran, 51
Dextrose, 51
Diet, 29
Dindevan, 61
Disinfection, 69
Dressings, 73
Dressing trolley, 74
Droplet infection, 19
Dust, 20
Dysphagia, 23
Dyspnoea, 30

Elderly, care of, 86
Electrolytes, 42
Embolism, pulmonary, 60
Emergencies, surgical, 81
Emphysema, surgical, 65
Epidural analgesia, 35
Epistaxis, 54
Epithelial tissue, 9
Erysipelas, 24
Escherichia coli, 17

Fistula, 64
Flies, 21
Fluid balance chart, 43
Frequency of urine, 86

Gas gangrene, 24
Gonococcus, 27
Gonorrhoea, 27
Granulation, 9
Gummata, 27

Haematemesis, 55
Haematoma, 5, 63
Haematuria, 55
Haemolytic streptococci, 16

Haemoptysis, 54
Haemorrhage, 53
Hartmann's solution, 51
Healing of wounds, 9
Heparin, 61
Hiccough, 57
Hutchinson's teeth, 27
Hygiene, in kitchen, 21
   personal, 18

Identity labels, 32, 84
Incised wounds, 5
Incontinence of urine, 86
Infarct, pulmonary, 61
Infection, 64
Inflammation, 12
Intensive Care Unit, 40
Intentional wounds, 4
Intra-cellular fluid, 42
Intravenous infusion, 47

Jewellery, 31

Keloid scarring, 7
Kifa clips, 78

Lacerations, 5
Largactil, 56
Lock-jaw, 22
Lumbar puncture, 36

Manitol, 51
Marzine, 56
Medial basilic vein, 48
Melaena, 55
Metabolism, 42
Michel's clips, 78
Micro-organisms, 16
Myobacterium, 25

Necrosis, 7
Neurogenic shock, 52
Non-pulmonary tuberculosis, 25
Non-touch technique, 75
Nutrition, 29

Obesity, 29
Observation of patient, 38

Oligaemic shock, 52
Ophthalmia neonatorum, 28
Orchitis, 27

Paralytic ileus, 58
Paresis, 62
Penicillin, 28
Pentothal, 34
Peritonitis, 62
Personal hygiene, 18
Plaster sores, 66
Plaster splint, 67
Pneumococcus, 12, 17
Post-operative care, 38
Pre-medication, 32
Pre-operative nursing, 30
Pulmonary,
  complications, 59
  embolism, 60
  infarct, 61
  tuberculosis, 25
Pulse, 38
Punctured wounds, 5
Pyaemia, 14

Recovery room, 40
Rectal injections, 34
Removal of, clips, 77
  stitches, 77
Respirations, 39
Retention of urine, 56
Retrovesical fistula, 64
Rhesus factor, 45

Ringer's solution, 51
Ryles tube, 40

Salpingitis, 27
Sanitary annexe, 20
Sepsis, 7, 69
Septicaemia, 13
Sequestrum, 7
Shock, 7, 52
Sinus, surgical, 7, 64
Skin, observation of, 39
  preparation of, 31
Sleep, 30
Sloughing, 7
Smoking, 30
Spinal analgesia, 35
Staphylococci, 12, 16
Sterilization, 69
Stitch abscess, 14
Stitches, removal of, 79
Streptococci, 12, 16
Streptomycin, 28
Suppository, 34
Suppuration, 7, 12
Surgical emergencies, 81
Syphilis, 26
Syphilitic ulcers, 14

Tetanus, 22
  prophylaxis, 23
Thrombosis, 61
Tourniquet, 54
Toxaemia, 13

Trauma, 4
Traumatic ulcers, 14
Treponema pallidum, 26
Trismus, 22
Trophic ulcers, 14
Tuberculosis, 25

Ulceration, 14
Ulcers,
  syphilitic, 14
  traumatic, 14
  trophic, 14
  varicose, 14
Urine, incontinence of, 86
  retention of, 56
Urticaria, 28

Varicose ulcers, 14
Venepuncture, 47
Venereal diseases, 36
Venesection, 49
Vomiting, 40, 56

Ward dressings, 72
Wounds,
  complications of, 7
  coverings, 77
  drainage of, 76
  healing of, 9
  intentional, 4
  rupture of, 63
  traumatic, 4
  types of, 4